FORENSIC ARCHAEOLOGY
AND HUMAN RIGHTS
VIOLATIONS

FORENSIC ARCHAEOLOGY AND HUMAN RIGHTS VIOLATIONS

Edited by

ROXANA FERLLINI, B.Sc., M.A., RFP

Co-ordinator M.Sc. Forensic Archaeological Science
Institute of Archaeology
University College London
London, United Kingdom

(With 15 Other Contributors)

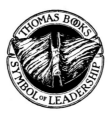

CHARLES C THOMAS • PUBLISHER, LTD.
Springfield • Illinois • U.S.A.

Published and Distributed Throughout the World by

CHARLES C THOMAS • PUBLISHER, LTD.
2600 South First Street
Springfield, Illinois 62704

© 2007 by CHARLES C THOMAS • PUBLISHER, LTD.

ISBN 978-0-398-07734-1 (hard)
ISBN 978-0-398-07735-8 (paper)

Library of Congress Catalog Card Number: 2006051293

Printed in the United States of America
UB-R-3

Library of Congress Cataloging-in-Publication Data

Forensic archaeology and human right violations / edited by Roxana Ferllini ;
   with 15 other contributors.
      p. cm.
   Includes bibliographical references and index.
   ISBN-13: 978-0-398-07734-1
   ISBN-10: 0-398-07734-7
   ISBN-13: 978-0-398-07735-8 (pbk.)
   ISBN-10: 0-398-07735-5 (pbk.)
      1. Forensic anthropology. 2. Forensic sciences. 3. Human remains (Arch-
   aeology) 4. Human rights. 5. Crimes against humanity. 6. Political atrocities.
   7. Crimes scenes. 8. Criminal investigations. 9. Medical jurisprudence. I.
   Ferllini, Roxana.

GN69.8.F64 2007
614'.17--dc22
                                                                      2006051293

To

Mark Goode for his never-ending support.

To

Professor Emeritus C. Melvin Aikens

of the University of Oregon

whose teaching and guidance gave me the opportunity

to discover the wonderful world of archaeology.

CONTRIBUTORS

Patricia Bernardi, Licda.
Forensic Anthropologist
Argentine Forensic Anthropology Team
Buenos Aires, Argentina
www.eaaf.org

John Cerone, B.S.E., J.D., LL.M.
Associate Professor of Law and Director
Center for International Law & Policy
New England School of Law
Boston, USA

Corrine Duhig, B.A. M.A. Ph.D. (CANTAB.) M.I.F.A.
Senior Lecturer
Faculty of Science and Technology
Anglia Ruskin University
Cambridge, United Kingdom

Peter Ellis M.A., M.B., BChir, FRCPA, MRACMA, FFFLM (UK)
Director of Forensic Medicine
Institute of Clinical Pathology and Medical Research,
Westmead, New South Wales
Australia

Roxana Ferllini, B.Sc., M.A., RFP
Co-ordinator M.Sc. Forensic Archaeological Science
Institute of Archaeology
University College London
London, United Kingdom

Luis Fondebrider, Lic.
Forensic Anthropologist
Argentine Forensic Anthropology Team
Buenos Aires, Argentina
www.eaaf.org

Ana María Gómez López, B.A., M.A.
Legal Representative and Community Relations Coordinator
EQUITAS, Equipo Colombiano Interdisciplinario de Trabajo Forense y Asistencia
Psicosocial.
(Colombian Interdisciplinary Team for Forensic Work and Psychosocial Services)
Bogotá, Colombia
www.equitas.org.co

John Hunter, B.A., Ph.D., MIFA, FSA, RFP
Professor of Ancient History and Archaeology
Institute of Archaeology and Antiquity
University of Birmingham
Birmingham, United Kingdom

Eva-Elvira Klonowski, M.Sc., Ph.D.
Senior Forensic Anthropologist
International Commission on Missing Persons
Sarajevo
Bosnia and Herzegovina

Kaisa Lalu, MD, Ph.D.
Senior Medical Examiner, Specialist in Forensic Medicine
State Provincial Office of Southern Finland
Helsinki, Finland

Andrés Patiño Umaña, B.A.
Forensic Anthropologist
Laboratory and Fieldwork Coordinator
EQUITAS, Equipo Colombiano Interdisciplinario de Trabajo Forense y Asistencia
Psicosocial.
(Colombian Interdisciplinary Team for Forensic Work and Psychosocial Services)
Bogotá, Colombia
www.equitas.org.co

Juha Rainio, MD, Ph.D.
Research Fellow
Institute of Legal Medicine
Catholic University of the Sacred Heart
School of Medicine
Rome, Italy

Antti Sajantila, MD, Ph.D.
Professor, Vice-Director
Department of Forensic Medicine
University of Helsinki
Helsinki, Finland

Barrie Simpson, B.A.(Hons), M.Sc. CertED
Hon. Research Fellow (Forensic Archaeology)
Institute of Archaeology and Antiquity
University of Birmingham,
Birmingham, United Kingdom

Mark Skinner, Ph.D., D.A.B.F.A.
Professor of Biological Anthropology
Department of Archaeology
Simon Fraser University
Burnaby
British Columbia, Canada

Mr. Ron Turnbull
Chief Security Advisor
UNICEF - Sudan
formerly
Head of Evidence Unit
International Criminal Tribunal for the former Yugoslavia
The Hague, Netherlands

PREFACE

The investigation of human rights abuses is becoming a more public and current issue on a global basis. Never before in recent memory has such a cross section of the world population been abused physically, emotionally, economically and militarily. Resultantly, vast areas of concern have been raised on the part of governmental and non-governmental agencies, human rights organizations, and also increasingly, interested members of the general public.

Open and rampant abuses directed against humanity fill our television screens and newspapers, and cross our daily thoughts and conversations. On a professional level, human rights workers and investigators have never been more necessary. As events unfold across the world, dedicated and often courageous professionals give of their time and expertise, in order to investigate such atrocities. This may place such individuals at odds with the motivations of the parties responsible for the issues that they are asked to analyze, often placing them at great personal risk.

There is also a higher purpose at stake with such work, which resides beyond the world of political and public opinion; the simple need for justice, healing and closure on the part of those who still remain after the fact, to mourn the needless loss of their loved ones. Human rights work in such circumstances should transcend the boundaries of mere conjecture and opinion. In its proper context and purest essence, such work should be intended to instil and nurture the healing process.

Forensic archaeology and forensic anthropology are now accepted as vital mechanisms in the machinery of investigating international human rights violations. It was with a wider perspective in mind that I decided to embark upon the production of this volume. I considered sincerely that there was, and still remains, a need for such issues to be brought into a more focused global context, in order to foster greater general understanding about the work that such professionals engage in, and the positive effect that their work can engender if approached with professionalism, and also the most vital element, personal sensitivity.

All the contributors to this volume live, or have worked in, areas of the world within situations that most individuals can scarcely imagine. The insights and work that they offer within this book is a testament to their skill, tenacity and courage. Progress, and working against the norms that we are often dealt with, does not come without risk. It is my sincere hope that those who learn and are inspired by the work of such individuals, contained within these pages, will take this to heart. Positive change truly does begin with understanding.

Roxana Ferllini
2007

ACKNOWLEDGMENTS

The creation of this volume would not have been possible without the valuable time and effort made by many fine contributors. By giving freely of their knowledge and experience, and weaving the same into the many pages they have written, valuable insights will be passed on to those interested in forensic archaeology and human rights issues. Also, to the many peer reviewers who gave unselfishly of their time to offer professional comments and suggestions, my sincere thanks.

To Mr. Stuart Laidlaw, photographer of the Institute of Archaeology, University College London, my sincere thanks for his professionalism and never-ending patience on countless occasions, when seeking his advice and technical support with the formatting of illustrations for this volume.

I wish to give my sincere thanks to Charles C Thomas, Publisher for providing the opportunity to develop this book, and for their valued and kind assistance during the maturation of the project.

Finally, I thank my husband Mark Goode, and my friends and colleagues who gave their constant support.

CONTENTS

FORENSIC ARCHAEOLOGY AND HUMAN RIGHTS VIOLATIONS

Chapter 1

HUMAN RIGHTS VIOLATIONS, PAST AND PRESENT: CONSEQUENCES AND INTERVENTIONS

Roxana Ferllini

BACKGROUND

On a global basis, contempt or violence has been directed, at one time or another, against civilian populations residing in many different countries and regions. Such behavior manifests itself in a variety of manners, and to different degrees, in part depending upon socio-cultural practices, political agendas and the interventions, or lack of, on the part of other nations. Such violations of human rights are varied in nature and occurrence, being evident under times of war, and also in periods of internal social turmoil. Resultantly, the methods by which such issues are investigated must be necessarily diverse, with a multi-disciplinary approach often being required in order to effectively complete the tasks at hand to the satisfaction of all parties. Such work may take place within the scope of a small community, involve a specific ethnic group or relatively few individuals, or be required on national scale. The consequences under investigation may be due to direct attacks against a specifically targeted group, or conversely, abuses meted out against innocent bystanders who may not be directly involved in such conflicts, but who still suffer as a result of the greater consequences, during or after the fact.

Perpetrators may choose to employ a variety of tactics in order to terrorize civilian populations; sexual assault is a common strategy (Zakir, 2003), involving the purposeful denigration of women by the means of rape. In many cases, the method of gang rape is chosen, and is often manifested in the unwilling presence of family members. Forced pregnancies are another tactic, resulting in the victims of such acts being shunned and stigmatized by their social group. Other consequences include the destruction of infrastructure and of private property, thereby effectively halting any possibility of continuing a meaningful daily existence. This latter tactic may compel those who are affected to be forced to survive under often protractedly extreme conditions. Such victims may suffer over considerable periods of time without adequate food, water, shelter, and also without the recourse of any manner of medical attention. In many cases, the injured may have survived initial abuses; however, for one reason or another after the fact, they subsequently succumb to starvation, disease, or from a lack of treatment to injuries that they may have sustained, creating in the process, a considerable pool of indirect deaths, separate from the initial event (Sandford, 2003). Such circumstances also serve to directly, or indirectly, cause the displacement of certain groups to different geographical areas, creating serious issues, not only for the refugees, but also creating turmoil and added pressures to host nations, many of which may also be experiencing their own internal problems, and often ill-equipped, or reluctant to deal with such added stresses. A case in point would be the massive exodus of refugees towards Goma in the Democratic Republic of the Congo (DRC), following the Rwandan genocide of 1994, which resulted in additional misery and suffering for those who had fled, and again, pressure on the part of the host nation. In the latter case, famine and disease resulted in the loss of approximately 30,000 lives, many of whom were buried en masse (Prunier, 2002).

Disappearances, forced detention, interrogation, torture, and summary executions that bypass any manner of legitimate judiciary procedure, may often be employed by the State against those considered to be its "enemies."

The deliberate displacement of children from their parents and common social group, or forcing that element of the population into armed conflict is another common type of human rights violation. As of 2004, it was estimated that approximately 30,000 children were involved within armed conflicts globally; many of them without recourse to any other option (Youth Advocate Programme International, 2004).

Armed conflicts take a toll not only on the targeted populations in question, but also create supplementary issues after the fact, such as residual land mines and other unexploded ordnance that remain in place across the territories in question. Such hazards must then be contended with long after former events have concluded, consequently causing the death or mutilation of innocent victims in times of "peace," and often rendering areas normally utilized for agriculture and other necessary activities to be highly reduced in scope. Contending with terror, intimidation and death casts a long shadow upon cultural, social and economic continuation. This often creates long-term psychological effects for those who were able to survive the initial process (Sack et al., 1999). As presented by Gómez López and Patiño Umaña in Chapter 8 of this volume, such persons, whether individual survivors or entire families, require much needed psychological assistance and sustained support in order to cope with the emotional scars left by the pain and suffering that they have sustained; however, some will continue to live in perpetual fear, often not being able to repair bonds of trust with respect to dealing with those in authority. The reconstruction of their lives becomes extremely challenging, due in part to the lack of the social and family network that they are accustomed to, and to the reduction of the community that they previously existed within.

When mass scale events transpire, a variety of changes will occur within affected communities, and also, in many cases, much farther afield. According to Sandford (2003) such modifications may be appreciated when conducting interviews with survivors, providing insights as to how the past and present are currently being perceived by a given population. Additionally, as a ramification of traumatic events, the language utilized to express their situation at any given moment in time is subject to change, that is, the language chosen may pass through a series of shifts with reference to the use of descriptive narrative that is chosen to describe and encode past events and present circumstances. Perceptions of self, family, community, and also future outlook are modified and expressed through such communication. New terms are often introduced, or the application of existing words or expressions, selected exclusively to express what has transpired by individuals who may have either suffered directly during possible atrocities, those who were indirectly affected, or persons who were relatively detached and distant observers to the events in question.

Some of the issues presented in this chapter may not pertain directly to those working in the field of forensic archaeology, or for other forensic specialists that become part of international missions that are convened to investigate the violation of human rights. Survivors of such acts will usually seek to locate their missing relatives, in order to commence, to some degree, the healing of their emotional wounds; ideally, this will contribute towards bringing a measure of closure to some of the issues that they shoulder. Victims of human rights abuses are also, by definition, one of the best sources of information pertaining to the actual events that occurred, and their eyewitness accounts are of crucial importance to many investigations (Sandford, 2003). Their contributions can also be of assistance when attempts are made to locate missing victims, and also with regard to participating in the identification process, as presented in Chapters 5 and 6 of this volume.

Acts as set forth above have not been unknown in past times. However, as the next section will illustrate, the past century stands as one of the most violent and grievous periods on record with reference to direction of violence against the innocent.

THE TWENTIETH CENTURY

In the context of modern history, the twentieth century will be acknowledged as an era characterized by a phenomenal increase in the frequency and magnitude of human rights violations against civilian populations. It was during the past century that humanity witnessed many different examples of such abuses, some state driven, some not, but often involving a blend of differing social, economic, political, civil, and religious spheres. In many instances, such violations were conducted systematically over time, contributing to the deliberate and calculated mass scale exterminations of entire populations. Such acts were a direct threat to life on an immediate level, but also served to negatively affect the quality of life and the integrity of socio-cultural groups after the fact. In some cases, the continued survival of certain cultural and ethnic groups lay in the balance, as total entities, and also on an individual level. It may be stated, therefore, that part of what characterizes the past century in relation to genocide is the inclusion and blending of race, religion, and territorial expansion. Perceptions also arose that certain social strata existing within a greater society that did not, in the opinion of the ruling classes, contribute effectively to society as a whole, could be legitimately eliminated, due to such rationalization (Kierman, 2003). However, such elements do not always work together at any given time, but on occasion, several factors and motivations may find themselves intertwined.

As explained by Cerone in Chapter 2, it was during this period of history when efforts were formally made, through the intervention of international law, to establish legal parameters in order to enforce sanctions against those who committed such crimes. No longer were such acts envisaged as being solely perpetrated by a faceless entity such as the State, but by individuals, who were to be held personally accountable for their own actions and motivations. Resultantly, this turning point spurred the creation of a variety of Tribunals and Courts since the conclusion of World War II, and most recently, the establishment of the International Criminal Court (ICC) in 2002, which is capable of overseeing cases on a global scale.

Initial Events

During World Wars I and II, events transpired that were without precedent in history. These acts were characterized by their sheer magnitude, and by the approaches taken by the states involved to effectively highjack the accepted norms of political and social behavior, in order to achieve their objectives.

In the early part of 1915, hundreds of Armenian leaders were killed by members of the Young Turks (who ruled the Ottoman Empire until the end of World War I), thereby paving the way to the first genocide of the twentieth century. These initial actions left the Armenian population defenseless, and totally vulnerable against what was to follow.

The First World War presented the Young Turks with the opportunity to conduct such killings in an organized manner, with the excuse that the Armenians were traitors to the Empire by siding with Russia (Mann, 2005). It is estimated that over one million of the Armenian population perished (Chorbajian, 1999; Rubinstein, 2004) through executions, slaughter, hunger, thirst, and disease. Others were affected by manner of deportation and displacement from their homes in the region of Anatolia (along the northeastern border with Russia), in the process often having to migrate to far-flung regions. Some were even forced into the Mesopotamian desert of Syria, where they died of exposure to the elements (Winter, 2003). Those Armenians who served in the army were purposefully gathered and placed into forced labor camps, where they eventually perished. These mass killings tailed off in 1918, once the Great War ended, only to resume again on a more limited scale, and finally concluding in 1923 with the fall of the Ottoman Empire (Hovannisian, 1992; Dadrian, 1995).

A prime example of the escalation of violence during the twentieth century was the killing of civilians at Nanking, popularly referred to as the "Rape of Nanking," at the hands of Imperial Japanese forces. The Japanese invasion was carried out during December of 1937, with the operation continuing for several weeks. Local populations were exterminated as Japanese troops gradually took control of the area. Their assaults were conducted at all hours of the day and night, and for weeks on end, including attacks on private and public premises, involving the rape of women of all ages, and murder by a variety of different means, including bayoneting. The death toll was estimated at 300,000 during the invasion; other Chinese regions were also affected in the same manner. China was not the only country which suffered high civilian casualties while under Japanese control; other areas included the Philippines, Borneo, the Moluccas (Indonesia), Singapore, the Solomon Islands and Hong Kong to name but a few (Lord Russell, 2002).

Another shaping event was perpetrated by the Nazi Third Reich from the late 1930s until the culmination of World War II. A fundamental ideological aim of the Nazi regime was the extermination of those who were not considered Aryan (the term employed by the Nazis to denote those of pure Germanic blood). Resultantly, the Jewish population was targeted for elimination, as were many other groups such as the Gypsies and Slavs. On another matter, the Nazis also wished to eliminate those who suffered from mental illnesses, or who exhibited any manner of hereditary abnormality, thereby adopting the principals of eugenics (Kierman, 2003).

In order to achieve their ideological aims, millions of persons were killed by the Nazi regime through the application of novel tactics. The Nazis were pragmatic and well-organized, and as such, the extermination procedures they elected to use were approached from an industrialized point of view. Logistics were set into place, a work force mobilized, and an infrastructure created which could effect the transportation and mass extermination of millions of individuals, and most importantly, provide for the efficient disposal of the bodies (Kierman, 2003; Weitz, 2003).

Ghettos were created in Eastern Europe in order to house those considered to be "sub-human." Concentration camps, such as Dachau and Mauthausen were employed to detain political "enemies" and any other individuals who were perceived as not being compliant with the ethos of the Nazi state (Engel, 2000:58; Wachsmann, 2004). However, not all were taken to concentration camps; alternatively, many individuals were transported directly to extermination centers, where those who were not listed for forced labor, or placed under medical experimentation, were put to death soon after their arrival (Engel, 2000).

Post World War II: A Continuation of Abuses

Although extreme examples of killing were witnessed during, and between, both World Wars, within China, nationalist repression during the Chinese civil war claimed an estimated 6 to 10 million lives between 1927 and 1949 (Valentino, 2004:83). From 1975 to 1979, the Cambodian population suffered under Pol Pot and the Khmer Rouge. Cambodia, referred to during the Pol Pot regime as Democratic Kampuchea, had its social fabric destroyed through a communist reformation of established social institutions, and by the implementation of an "autarchic agrarian regime" (Shawcross, 2002:39; Weitz, 2003), which displaced the urban population into rural areas. During this process, it is estimated that well over two million Cambodians perished, including children and the elderly, through forced labor, starvation and disease. Many were tortured and executed because they were perceived to be enemies of the state (Zakir, 2003; Rubinstein, 2004).The situations in East Timor after the Indonesian military invasion (by the Tentara Nasional Indonesia forces, TNI) from 1975 to 1999 (until the intervention of the United Nations), and that of Somalia from 1988 to 1991 resulted in an estimated 100-200,000 and 50-60,000 individuals perishing respectively, due to the effects of counter-guerrilla mass killings alone (Valentino, 2004:83), further illustrating a continuation of brutal actions directed against civilians.

Perhaps one of the most alarming events to occur in recent times was the Rwandan genocide of 1994, which lasted 100 days. The victims were mainly Tutsi and some Hutu, the latter being those who disagreed with the extermination of the former, and who had elected to come to their aid. In spite of the relatively short time frame in which it occurred, unprecedented events transpired. For example, women killed their own husbands and children, neighbors turned against each other, classmates murdered one another, teachers and school officials savaged their co-workers and pupils, and doctors and nurses turned against their patients. Those who sought refuge in hospitals were turned in to be disposed of (the sick, wounded or plainly hiding), and pregnant women, or those who just had given birth, and their newborns, were hacked to death with machetes, or killed by other means, along with other hospital patients. Many members of the clergy turned against their parishioners by refusing to assist, or by turning them over to the authorities; some nuns and priests were murdered for not wishing to participate. Following the conclusion of events in Rwanda, The International Criminal Tribunal for Rwanda (ITCR)was convened during November 1994, under the Chapter VIII of the Charter of the United Nations. The Rwandan genocide was considered to be one of, if not the most, intense genocides of modern times (African Rights, 1995; Prunier, 2002; Ferllini, 1999; Zakir, 2003).

At the time of writing, there are still many situations in process in which mass killings are taking place, such as the case of the Sudan. The conflict within the Sudan commenced in 2003 in the Darfur region, within the western sector of that country. The estimated number of casualties is not firmly known; however it is believed that many thousands have been killed, raped, tortured and displaced from their homes by governmental forces, and by the Janiawid faction (Arab Muslim group), (Amnesty International, 2006; Johnson, 2003; Prunier, 2005).

FORENSIC ARCHAEOLOGY: INITIAL INTERVENTIONS

Initial interventions of forensic archaeology in the investigation of human rights abuses were conducted in Latin America, commencing in the 1980s. This region has witnessed a series of gross human rights violations. A brief description of the social context and developments will be provided, as such elements are connected to events and attitudes that lead to the abuses against civilian populations in most areas of the region.

From a historical perspective, Latin America has suffered through many acts of brutality, initially perpetrated against its indigenous populations, commencing during the late 1400s by European conquerors during the *conquista*; throughout the colonial period, the position of the indigenous populations continued to decline, and they were effectively subjugated to an inferior status. During the past century, civilian populations from many of the nations which compose this part of the world have suffered violations inflicted upon them by their own governmental authorities, and in particular, military interventions. A vast majority of the large-scale abuses were perpetrated during the 1970s and 1980s, stemming from movements that began decades before, or resulting from long-rooted historical issues. However, independent of the particular reasons or rationales, the toll inflicted on human life has been immense, and the legacy to be dealt with by for those who survive may often be insurmountable.

For these developing nations, socio-economic problems and abuse towards civilians has been a part of the everyday landscape for many decades. The military establishments of most countries have taken over the direct control of numerous aspects of the every day running of society. According to Kruijt and Koonings (2004:18), there are four areas that the military strives to manage in order to exert its influence effectively:

1. The control of intelligence
2. Predominance over police forces
3. The control of local and regional development (many remote areas remain under the sole care of the military)
4. Total immunity on a legal level, thereby being able to abuse with impunity.

Another important factor to consider in the equation is the plethora of paramilitary forces that have arisen from different backgrounds, as witnessed in Argentina, Chile, Colombia and Mexico. Abuses carried out by such groups in counter-insurgency capacities have been manifested in countries such as El Salvador and Guatemala. Such organizations often work hand-in-hand with government death squads, in order to force the civilian population into compliance by the use of terror and murder (Kruijt and Koonings, 2004).

Individual states that maintain a strong military presence often exhibit an endemic element of corruption within the military itself, the effects of which then trickle down to subsequently taint their respective governmental bureaucracies and judicial systems. However, the removal of military dictatorships, and the introduction of more open and "democratic" systems has also led to the creation of new problems, including internationally organized criminal activity. One of the by products of such businesses is the illegal narcotics trade, which has served to fuel violence against, and create misery for, the peasant communities within the countries where the drugs are produced. A prime example would be coca production within the Andean region of South America, which provides raw materials for the cocaine trade (Koonings and Kruijt, 2004). In essence, levels of violence have actually risen with the introduction of democratization, partly due to the huge amount of power that is available solely to a relatively tiny proportion of the elite class. Such changes, brought about under the pretence of democratization, do not benefit the poor, who are on the increase in numbers within such developing nations. Also increasing are patterns of continuing human rights abuses, which are often typical of previous eras of dictatorship and militarism. Resultantly, the general populations often perceive themselves as isolated and powerless. Many sectors of the societies in question suffer constantly from the lack of access to basic human requirements, such as potable water and adequate shelter (Kruijt and Koonings, 1999).

South America

South American nations have for the most part experienced intense oppression brought on by dictatorships, creating a climate of fear and persecution for those considered enemies of the state. Of particular interest to this volume is the persecution, disappearances, torture and killings of those in Argentina and Chile commencing in the 1970s.

In the case of Argentina, a three-man junta was installed, headed by army general J. R. Videla, resulting from a military coup that occurred during the early part of 1976. The regime continued until 1983, and during its seven-year rule, many civilians were abducted and transported to one of the hundreds of detention centers scattered throughout the country, where those individuals were tortured, and most were subsequently executed. The bodies were disposed of in a variety of manners, including covert burial in public cemeteries (Joyce and Stover, 1991). Such events were everyday occurrences during the *Guerra Sucia.*

During this era of terror, women searching for their missing children would congregate at the Plaza de Mayo, a landmark in the capital city of Buenos Aires, demanding answers as to the whereabouts of their loved ones. Over time, they formed a non-governmental group, the Grandmothers of the Plaza de Mayo, which actively pursued justice for the missing. In 1983, with the establishment of a democratic government, a priority was established for locating the thousands of individuals who had disappeared and perished under the previous military regime.

As a result of these events, interventions by the families of the missing, and the organizations created by them. The National Commission on the Disappeared of Persons (CONADEP) was created by the newly established government, which made appeals for information in order to locate those who had disappeared. Consequently, judicial personnel agreed to the exhumation of hundreds of NN (no name) graves. The initial methods utilized were utilitarian in nature, not being precise and detail oriented as would be the case if forensic archaeology was being formally practiced. This crude process produced a public outcry, as the excavations were actually serving to destroy many finds, and valuable forensic evidence was being lost. Resultantly, assistance was requested from the American Association for the Advancement of Science (AAAS), as it was evident that the capacity to process the data and recover the remains did not exist at that time within Argentina. In 1984, a delegation of American forensic scientists travelled to Argentina; among them was forensic anthropologist Dr. Clyde Snow. Resultantly, the Argentine Forensic Anthropology Team (EEAF) was created (further elaborated by Bernardi and Fondebrider in Chapter 9, of this volume) in order to fulfill the greater objective independently, where upon work proceeded in a structured and scientific manner, and does so to the present day (Joyce and Stover, 1991; EAAF, 2005a).

Within Chapter 9 of this book, the problems posed when archaeology and anthropology was initially applied within the context of human rights investigations is presented. Additionally, that account also exemplifies the importance of effective historical research as a vital consideration prior to the commencement of the search, location and recovery of individuals, with special reference to those who had disappeared, and who had been covertly buried in public cemeteries as NNs.

In 1973, General Augusto Pinochet came to power in Chile after the elected president, Salvador Allende, was assassinated during a coup; the incoming regime created a wave of terror and repression in order to pacify the Chilean public (Burbach, 2003). Here, in a similar fashion, a section of the public was also targeted, abducted, and faced a similar fate in detention centers as would the Argentinan population a few years later. As no warrants or judicial procedures existed or were required, thousands simply disappeared (Ensalaco, 2000:89). The objective was to eliminate individuals who were considered likely to cause problems for the regime, such as those labeled as being in agreement with leftist ideologies, any manner of political opponents, and anyone who might potentially disagree with any aspect of the regime. Individuals were rounded up throughout the country; these acts became popularly known as the "Caravans of Death"; others, in their naivety, voluntarily surrendered themselves at military posts (Burbach, 2003: 48; Ensalaco, 2000:84).

These operations were coordinated by the Directorate for National Intelligence (DINA), which was charged with overseeing the kidnappings, the workings of the detention centers (such as the National Stadium in the capital Santiago, and others created by the intelligence agency), the logistics, interrogation procedures, classification of detainees, and the processing of intelligence. Those who immediately resisted were often summarily executed. In the case of detainees, most were eliminated and disposed of by a variety of different methods (Ensalaco, 2000:55). The concealment and burial of the bodies was conducted in part in clandestine graves, ravines, and by dumping them in disused wells and mines. Instances occurred in which detainees were drugged up, taken in a helicopter, and once over the Pacific Ocean, after having their stomachs slashed to prevent their bodies from floating, were thrown into the water (Ensalaco, 2000:94). The survivors of this violent era were seriously affected psychologically, and most citizens knew of someone who had gone missing (Ensalaco, 2000:95). Although the exact number of those killed during the Pinochet regime is unknown, it is estimated that over 3,000 individuals disappeared; many others chose to go into exile (Burbach, 2003).

Following the Argentinian model, in due course, the Chilean Forensic Anthropology Group (GAF) was created in the late 1980s; many of the missing were successfully located, and subsequently identified.

With reference to Colombia, this country has suffered through phenomenal levels of human rights abuses and extra judicial murders. Continuous outrages have been perpetrated by the army, right-wing paramilitaries, leftist-guerillas, and the police, amongst other numerous players. When the ongoing process of globalization are also added to the picture, the outlook for Colombia's long-suffering population appears very fragile indeed. The effects of such cycles of violence in Colombia, with insights pertaining to ongoing efforts to locate and identify those who have succumbed as a result of that country's prolonged internal strife, is treated in detail within Chapter 8 of this volume.

Central America

As in the case of South America, oppression brought on by dictatorships, and the abuse handed out on the part of the ruling elite has cast a serious toll on the lives of the Central American populations. Most countries have at some juncture witnessed waves of violence directed towards civilians, mainly focused against the much oppressed and poor peasant classes. The latter group were particularly targeted, as they were considered to be an integral potential element of revolutions, and as such, were instinctively branded as "leftists." The poorest populations within Central America have suffered severely due to governmental corruption, and have often paid a high price in lives as a result of the acts of intimidation directed against them. Guatemala is probably one of the hardest hit nations in the area, with a long history of ethnic violence towards its Mayan population. From the mid-1950s onwards, Guatemalans went into confrontation with the military, due to civil unrest, thereby opening the door to guerrilla intervention. The guerrilla movement presented an option of opposition for various groups, such as farmers, unions and peasants, but there was a high price to be paid; during the last 30 years, the civil war in Guatemala has caused tens of thousands of deaths, with as many again listed as "disappeared." Hundreds of villages were destroyed, and the inhabitants massacred; an estimated 1.5 million are believed to have been displaced, and over 100,000 have fled to Mexico. The victims were over 80 percent Maya, the rest being ladino, those of Indian and European mix. Because of such a high degree of violence towards the Mayan population, that particular group has been decimated by massacres perpetrated against it on a continual basis, over many years (Sandford, 2003:148; Kruijt and Koonings 1999). During the early 1990s, the Guatemalan Forensic Anthropology Team (EAFG) came into existence. This organization, known today as the Guatemalan Forensic Anthropology Foundation (FAFG), is actively involved in the search, recovery, and identification of the victims. Up until 2006, the FAFG has conducted over 500 investigations, and many thousands of bodies have been recovered (FAFG, 2006).

El Salvador is another nation within the region that suffered through persistent violence during the 1970s. In the 1980s it was still experiencing civil unrest and guerrilla confrontations, wherein a social revolution took place. Such consciousness was brought on in part by the clergy and religious activists, with several groups being created to fight against social injustice; in turn, death squads commenced a campaign of terror throughout the country. Between 1980 and 1982, violations of human rights were at such high levels that El Salvador was "put on the map" in recognition of the intensity of major human rights infractions that were occurring there. Estimates indicate that more than 60,000 individuals were killed as a result of armed confrontations, including national and foreign religious personnel, and also international aid workers. Thousands were forced out of their homes, and most of those who migrated overseas moved to the US (Byrne, 1996). The massacre perpetrated at El Mozote is a vivid example of the manner by which such atrocities were committed by the military against the peasant class, as an act of oppression and intimidation towards the guerrillas. In December 1981, the army marched into El Mozote hamlet, and ordered the inhabitants to the central square. There, the population was divided, and taken to various buildings where many were murdered and decapitated. Young women were taken into the hills, where they were raped and then killed. Others were forced to march into the countryside, where they were later gunned down. Children did not escape the attentions of the soldiers, and most of the community's infrastructure was destroyed, a pattern conforming to that observed in other areas of the country, with the larger objective of impeding those in the countryside from being able to make a living. Rural populations were also caught in the cross-fire when the armed forces were searching for guerrillas (Binford, 1996; Dutton et al., 2005).

Nearly eleven years after the massacre at El Mozote, forensic archaeologists from the Argentine Forensic Anthropology Team (EEAF) conducted excavations in the area, recovering a minimum of 143 incomplete skeletonized individuals, and documenting other important evidence in the process (Binford, 1996:127; EAAF, 2006). Also possible as a result of their work, was the reconstruction of some of the events that had transpired during the massacre. The data collected was subsequently presented to the Truth Commission, set up by the United Nations (Binford, 1996).

Such examples illustrate the evolution and foundation of forensic archaeology and forensic anthropology as distinct disciplines, to be applied routinely in any investigation of human rights violations, when the recovery and identification of the victims is necessary. These interventions have increased through the years, and presently, as a matter of course, any mission involved in such investigative work will include such professionals. Work being performed by a few individuals is no longer acceptable, with tasks now being shared as part of full a multi-disciplinary intervention.

INTERNATIONAL AWARENESS

Since the 1980s, forensic participation in human rights investigations has increased markedly. Such interventions have occurred in widespread areas of the world including (and aside from those already mentioned above) Perú, Honduras, East Timor, the Philippines, Sierra Leone, Democratic Republic of the Congo (DRC), Zimbabwe, Ethiopia, Haiti, Sri Lanka, and Cyprus (EAAF, 2005b).

When participating in such international missions, the personal risk to those involved in the field may be high; the threat of unexploded ordnance, terrorism and other forms of violence are realistic factors to consider. It is for this reason, as presented in Chapters 3 and 4, that team organization and effective management of security should be taken seriously, and put effectively into action. Hunter and Simpson offer in Chapter 11 an account of the dangers and challenges of working within a war zone, and how the cooperation of military personnel in providing security is a must for human rights workers on the ground.

Additionally, the work to be accomplished in the field and at mortuary should ideally be coordinated by individuals with experience of the tasks at hand, as presented by Duhig and Turnbull in Chapter 4. However, an important additional element of any effective outcome will involve the careful prior procurement and coordination of equipment, and an accurate awareness of the locally available infrastructure, also covered in Chapter 3.

Many organizations have formed internationally which assist with the investigation and aftermath of such crimes and abuses; such bodies may be inter-governmental and non-governmental in nature. The intervention of non-governmental organizations (NGOs) as independent monitoring bodies, such as Amnesty International, Human Rights Watch and other groups, has been of vital assistance, creating a public focus and international awareness of human rights issues. NGOs may exist as both national and foreign entities, in the latter case, their presence, either on a constant or intermittent basis provides a neutral point of contact within areas of conflict, and their length of stay in trouble spots may often be lengthy. In either case, their interventions are often associated with close ties to local organizations (May, 2005; Burbach, 2003).

The effects of globalization have seeped into most elements and aspects of everyday living. National and popular culture, economics, politics, and socio-political trends, among others, are all influenced by this phenomenon. Also included within the modern global view are human rights issues. The growing persistence of such abuses is now being manifested as a large sphere of influence with reference to the shaping of world events. With the advent of the mass media and the 24/7 approach to television reporting, the availability of cable channels dedicated exclusively to news reporting, and with access to the Internet on the increase, it is almost impossible not to be aware of situations occurring across the world in "real time" (Burbach, 2003; Kishan and Freedman, 2003).

Even after considerable periods of time have elapsed, rival political views, and sustained support for accused parties may resurface. This can create tensions between those in favor of justice, and those who might have vested interests to oppose it. Such an example of this would be the arrest, during 1998, of Chilean General A. Pinochet in London, England (Silva, 1999). Human rights activists, and those who had suffered under his regime, saw that event as a landmark victory, while many of his supporters, in Chile, and abroad, were outraged and claimed injustice.

CURRENT CONCERNS

At present, forensic archaeology and forensic anthropology are being applied in areas where conflicts have occurred and where victim location and identification of bodies is requested.

An example of investigative work being conducted on events that have occurred recently is that in process within the Balkan region of Eastern Europe, where abuses initiated during the early1990s have received immense political and media attention. The region descended into a war which eventually led to ethnic cleansing, resulting in the deaths of tens of thousands of civilians, many of whose sole offence had been belonging to the wrong religious or ethnic affiliation; there was also a high displacement of the population into neighboring regions (Booth, 2001; Weitz, 2003). Mass rape and other types of sexual assault took place; such tactics became a weapon of war. Women who resultantly became pregnant brought shame to their families and communities, thereby indirectly assisting the further disintegration of their culture, the intended objective of the perpetrators.

Human rights abuses occurred within the Balkans on a vast and apparently structured basis. Many of the victims were concealed by guilty parties in inaccessible situations, such as within mines and caves, creating great difficulties for human rights investigators with respect to recovering the remains in question (Klonowski, 2007). Also troubling was the fact that media coverage of the Balkan conflict extended over many years, with many inexcusable events being witnessed virtually live within media coverage.

An issue to consider in connection with the situation that occurred within the former Yugoslavia, was that such gross abuses were openly taking place literally on the doorstep of Europe. Concentration camps were envisaged at that time as being a dark element of Europe's recent historical past, but the world was again presented with the nightmarish images of gaunt and brutalized individuals, detained behind barbed wire fences. The complex and convoluted political situation extant in the region presents its own unique challenges while attempts are made to investigate human rights abuses that occurred there; pertinent observations of the same, and the extensive work undertaken to investigate and identify victims within the Balkans is presented in Chapter 7 of this volume by Klonowski.

The current situation in Afghanistan is a testament to the effects of decades of social and political upheaval, exacerbated by prolonged and brutal armed conflicts, which has resulted in the direct and indirect deaths of millions of individuals. Afghanistan's history has passed through many different periods of political control and change. In 1979, the Soviet Union, with the backing of the then existing government, invaded the country. Organized resistance was directed against them on the part of different groups, including the Islamic freedom fighters, referred to popularly as the Mujahideen (holy muslim warriors). At that juncture in its history, Afghanistan was caught within a clash of opposing Cold War ideologies (Amnesty International, 1995; Misra, 2004); with elements opposing the government being supported and funded by the CIA and other interests.

Following the Soviet withdrawal from Afghanistan in 1989, the existing government collapsed after internal military elements conspired against it, whereupon Afghanistan was declared an Islamic State. The country was in a state of chaos, and the situation continued to slide into further decline; armed conflicts continued amongst internal factions struggling for political power, and violations of human rights persisted (Amnesty International, 1995:8; Rasanayagam, 2003). In the mid-1990s, the Taliban (a movement of religious scholars and former Mujahideen) eventually took control of most of the country. Shari'ah (Islamic Law) was enforced, which heavily suppressed the human rights and freedoms of the population. Cruel punishments, public floggings and amputations meted out to the non-compliant were commonplace (Amnesty International, 1998). The rival political entity to the Taliban, the Northern Alliance, a coalition of warlords which currently control different sectors of the country (Human Rights Watch, 2003) are also accused of killing members of the Taliban.

The obvious difficulties involved in the undertaking of meaningful human rights work in such a hostile political and social climate as exists in Afghanistan speak for themselves; however, a rare and meaningful insight can be obtained through the experiences of Skinner, contained in Chapter 10.

The most pressing human rights issue of the initial years of the twenty-first century is the continued turmoil within Iraq. As a result of armed conflict and insurgency, many thousands of civilian deaths have been caused. Since the commencement of the US led invasion of 2003, the country has been in the forefront of media attention. Human rights violations inflicted upon the Iraqi people by its former government, under the dictatorship of Saddam Hussein, have been well-documented, and form an open element of the history of that country.

Specific ethnic entities within Iraq were targeted by the former government, such as the Kurdish and Marsh Arab populations. In the past, the Kurds have endured, in addition to human rights violations, the ransacking and destruction of their lands and villages. Perhaps one of the most severe attacks against the Iraqi Kurdish population occurred during 1987 and 1988, while Iraq was losing its footing in the war it was waging against Iran. Afraid that the Kurdish population was supporting and joining the pershmergas (groups of Kurdish fighters), operations were carried out against them by the Iraqi military, resulting in the looting and destruction of thousands of villages. Iraqi Kurds also endured chemical weapon attacks, again directed against them by the Iraqi military. A chemical assault upon the town of Halabja, situated near the Iranian border, and considered to be a peshmerga stronghold, received media attention, and international condemnation, and is believed to have killed approximately 5,000 civilians (a conservative figure). Forensic investigations, through exhumations, body analysis and environmental sampling to verify the use of chemical weapons, were conducted in 1992 by Physicians for Human Rights (PHR, a Boston-based non-governmental organization) (PHR, 1993).

The recent discovery of large scale mass graves within Iraq indicates that extra-judicial killings appear to have been conducted. According to Yildiz and Blass (2003:176), 300,000 Kurds are believed to be concealed within these graves. This situation has created the necessity of investigating the locations in question formally, in order to accurately verify what has transpired.

Investigations conducted by forensic archaeologists within Iraq have already begun, as is effectively illustrated in Chapter 11. However, at the time of writing, the security situation in Iraq has declined markedly, and resultantly, productive work cannot reasonably be expected to occur to any large degree until the internal conflict that has taken hold since the occupation of that country has abated.

CONCLUSIONS

This chapter illustrates past and present issues related to global human rights abuses. Results obtained from the investigations of such events are never predictable, as many variables are apt to occur that may affect performance in the field.

Forensic archaeology and anthropology are vital tools in the investigative process, assisting with the recovery of the victims and associated evidence, and arriving at identifications when possible. As a result of such work, documentation is gathered that will permit the guilty parties to be more effectively prosecuted through relevant national and international legal bodies.

REFERENCES

African Rights (1995). *Rwanda not so innocent: When women become killers.* London: African Rights.

Amnesty International (1995). Afghanistan: International responsibility for human rights. http://web.amnesty.org/library/index/engASA110091995 Accessed August 20, 2006.

Amnesty International (1998). Afghanistan flagrant abuse of the right to life and dignity. http://web.amnesty.org/library/Index/engASA110031998 Accessed August 20, 2006.

Amnesty International (2006). Sudan crying out for safety. http://web.amnesty.org/library/Index/ENGAFR540552006. Accessed 5 October, 2006.

Binford, L. (1996). *The El Mozote massacre: Anthropology and human rights.* Tucson: The University of Arizona Press.

Booth, K. (Ed.) (2001). *The Kosovo tragedy: The human rights dimensions.* London: Frank Cass Publishers.

Burbach, R. (2003). *The Pinochet affair: State terrorism and global justice.* London: Zed Books.

Byrne, H. (1996). *El Salvador's civil war: Study of revolution.* London: Lynne Rienner Publishers, Inc.

Chorbajian, L. (1999). Introduction. In *Studies in comparative genocide*, Chorbajian, L., and Shirinian, G. (Eds.). London: Macmillan Press Ltd., pp. xv-xxxv.

Dadrian, V. (1995). The history of the Armenian genocide: Ethnic conflict from the Balkans to Anatolia to the Caucasus. Oxford: Berghan Books.

Dutton, D., Boyanowsky, E., and Bond, M. (2005). Extreme mass homicide: From military massacre to genocide. *Aggression and Violent Behavior, 10:* 437–473.

EAAF website (2005a). http://eaaf.typepad.com/founding_of_eaaf/. Accessed July 19, 2006.

EAAF website (2005b). http://www.eaaf/org/reports/index.php Accessed July 19. 2006.

EAAF website (2006). http://www.eaaf.org/reports/elsalvador.php Accessed July 19, 2006.

Engel, D. (2000). *The Holocaust: The Third Reich and the Jews.* Harlow: Pearson Education Limited.

Ensalaco, M. (2000). *Chile under Pinochet: Recovering the truth.* Philadelphia: University of Philadelphia Press.

FAFG website (2006). http://www.fafg.org/ Accessed July 17, 2006.

Ferllini, R. (1999). The role of forensic antropology in human rights issues. In Forensic Osteological Analysis: ABook of Case Studies, Fairgrieve, S. (Ed.). Springfield: Charles C Thomas, pp. 287-302.

Hovannisian, R. (Ed.) (1992). *The Armenian genocide.* London: Macmillan Academic and Professional, LTD.

Human Rights Watch (2003). Afghanistan: Warlords implicated in new abuses. http://hrw.org/press/2003/07/afghan072903.htm Accessed August 20, 2006.

Johnson, D. (2003). *The root causes of Sudan's civil wars.* Kampala: Fountain Publishers, 2003.

Joyce, C., and Stover, E. (1991). *The stories bones tell: Witnesses from the grave.* New York: Ballantine Books.

Kierman, B. (2003). The modernity of genocide: War, race, and revolution in the twentieth century. In *The specter of genocide: Mass murder in historical perspective*, Gellately, R., and Kierman, B. (Eds.). Cambridge: Cambridge University Press, pp. 29–51.

Kishan, D., and D. Freedman (Eds.) (2003). *War and the media: Reporting conflict 24/7.* London: Sage Publications.

Klonowski, E. (2007). Exhumations in Bosnia and Herzegovina: Caves as mass graves, from recovery to identification. In *Forensic anthropology: Case studies from Europe*, Brickley, M., and Ferllini, R. (Eds.). Springfield: Charles C Thomas. In press.

Koonings, K., and Kruijt, D. (Eds.) (2004). *Armed actors: Organized violence and State failure in Latin America.* London: Zed Books Ltd.

Kruijt, D., and Kroonings, K. (1999). Introduction: Violence and fear in Latin America. In *Societies of fear: The legacy of civil war, violence and terror in Latin America*, Koonings, K., and Kruijt, D. (Eds.). London: Zea Books, Ltd., pp. 1-30.

Kruijt, D., and Koonings, K. (2004). The military and their shadowy brothers. In *Armed actors: Organized violence and State failure in Latin America*, Koonings, K., and Kruijt, D. (Eds.) London: Zed Books, Ltd., pp. 16–32.

Lord Russell of Liverpool (2002). *The knights of Bushido: A short history of Japanese war crimes*. London: Greenhill Books.

Mann, M. (2005). *The dark side of democracy: Explaining ethnic cleansing*. Cambridge: Cambridge University Press.

May, R. (2005). Human Rights NGOs and the role of civil society in democratization. In *(Un)civil Societies: Human rights and democratic transitions in Eastern Europe and Latin America*, May, R.A., and Milton, A.K. (Eds.). Oxford: Lexington Books, pp. 1–10.

Misra, M. (2004). *Afghanistan: The Labyrinth of Violence*. Cambridge: Polity Press.

PHR website (1993). Nerve gas used in Northern Iraq on Kurds. http://www.phrusa.org/research/chemical_weapons/chemiraqgas2.html Accessed August 20, 2006.

Prunier, G. (2002). *The Rwandan crisis: History of a genocide*. London: C. Hurst & Company.

Prunier, G. (2005). *Darfur: The ambiguous genocide*. London: Hurst & Company.

Rasanayagam, A. (2003). *Afghanistan: A modern history*. New York: I. B. Tauris & Co., Ltd.

Rubinstein, W.D. (2004). *Genocide: A history*. Edinburgh: Pearson Educational Limited.

Sack, W., Him, C., and Dickason, D. (1999). Twelve-year follow-up study of Khmer youths who suffered massive trauma as children. *J. American Academy of Child & Adolescent Psychiatry, 38*(9): 1173–1179.

Sandford, V. (2003). *Buried secrets: Truth and human rights in Guatemala*. New York: Palgrave Macmillan.

Shawcross, W. (2002). Lessons of Cambodia. In *The new killing fields: Massacre and the politics of intervention*, Mills, N., and Brunner, K. (Eds.). New York: Basic Books, pp. 37–49.

Silva, P. (1999). Collective memories, fears and consensus: the political psychology of Chilean democratic transition. In *Societies of fear: The legacy of civil war, violence and terror in Latin America*, Koonings, K. and Kruijt, D. (Eds.). London: Zea Books, Ltd., pp. 171-196.

Valentino, B.A. (2004). *Final solutions: Mass killing and genocide in the 20th century*. New York: Cornell University Press.

Wachsmann, N. (2004). *Hitler's prisons: Legal terror in Nazi Germany*. New Haven: Yale University Press.

Weitz, E.D. (2003). *A century of genocide: Utopias of race and nations*. Princeton: Princeton University Press.

Winter, J. (2003). Under the Cover of War: The Armenian genocide in the context of total war. In *The specter of genocide: Mass murder in historical perspective*, Gellately, R., and Kierman, B. (Eds.). Cambridge: Cambridge University Press, pp. 189–213.

Yildiz, K., and Blass, T. (2003). *The Kurds in Iraq: The past, present and future*. London: Kurdish Human Rights Project.

Youth Advocate Programme International (YAP International) (2004). http://www.yapi.org/conflict/. Accessed August 2, 2006.

Zakir, M. (2003). *Human rights, crimes against humanity and State terror*. Leicester: Zap-Critique Books.

Chapter 2

THE NATURE OF INTERNATIONAL CRIMINAL LAW AND IMPLICATIONS FOR INVESTIGATIONS

JOHN CERONE

INTRODUCTION

Violations of international criminal law are rarely committed in isolation. Frequently, they are perpetrated in the context of a broader project or a massive upheaval consisting of numerous such violations. The context and scale of these events can create numerous logistical difficulties in conducting investigations. As described by the US government in preparation for the 1945 Yalta Conference:

> [T]he crimes to be punished have been committed upon such a large scale that the problem of identification, trial and punishment of their perpetrators presents a situation without parallel in the administration of criminal justice. In thousands of cases, it will be impossible to establish the offender's identity or to connect him with the particular act charged. Witnesses will be dead, otherwise incapacitated and scattered. The gathering of proof will be laborious and costly, and the mechanical problems involved in uncovering and preparing proof of particular offenses one of appalling dimensions.[1]

Overcoming such difficulties can consume massive amounts of human, temporal, and material resources. However, in addition to these

---

1. Memorandum to President Roosevelt from the Secretaries of State and War and the Attorney General ("Yalta Memorandum"), January 22, 1945, at http://www.yale.edu/lawweb/avalon/imt/jackson/jack01.htm.

practical difficulties, other difficulties stem from the law to be applied in such cases.

There are three categories of crimes at the core of international criminal law that fall within the jurisdiction of international criminal courts – war crimes, genocide, and crimes against humanity. The legal nature of these crimes will often require proof of legal elements that pose an additional burden on investigators. In order to understand these legal requirements, it is essential to understand the nature and substance of international criminal law.[2]

INTRODUCTION TO INTERNATIONAL CRIMINAL LAW

Central to a proper understanding of international criminal law is the fact that it is a discrete body of public international law and, as such, operates in the context of the international legal system. At the same time, the character of international criminal norms, as norms capable of engaging the criminal responsibility of individual human beings, is distinct from that of most other norms of public international law.

Public International Law

From the inception of the Westphalian system, the sovereign equality of states and the related principle of non-intervention were paramount. As a horizontal system, where sovereign states were horizontally juxtaposed with no higher authority, its substantive norms consisted of a network of reciprocal obligations that focused almost exclusively on interstate relations.[3] Norms generated within this system have been traditionally

---

2. Generally, the phrase "international criminal law" may refer to a variety of international norms, including those governing such matters as extradition and mutual cooperation in law enforcement and judicial proceedings. In this chapter, the phrase is used in its strict sense – it refers to that body of norms of public international law the breach of which will give rise to individual criminal responsibility.

3. Another consequence of this horizontal structure is the consent-based nature of international law. As sovereign equals, all states are of equal legal status, and thus may only be bound by obligations that they have created or chosen to accept. While this voluntarist model was altered following World War II and the adoption of the Charter of the United Nations, the international legal system still rests on the principle of state sovereignty and any legal analysis must begin with this principle. The sources of international law, reflecting this requirement of state consent, are treaties, custom, and general principles of law. Statute of the International Court of Justice, art. 38.

understood to have as their legal subject the state alone, and their breach gave rise only to the responsibility of the state. Individual human beings could only be bound by international law indirectly, if at all.

The Evolution of International Criminal Law

The horrors of the Second World War spawned a host of developments in international law. Among the most significant was the crystallization of the principle that violation of certain norms of international law could give rise to individual criminal responsibility. According to this principle, certain serious violations of international law would engage not only the classical form of responsibility in international law, i.e., the responsibility of the state, but also that of the individual human beings perpetrating the violation. Such perpetrators could be criminally prosecuted and punished for these violations of international law.

The emergence of this principle was primarily driven by the need to develop effective means of enforcement. As reasoned by the International Military Tribunal at Nuremberg, "Crimes against international law are committed by men, not by abstract entities, and only by punishing individuals who commit such crimes can the provisions of international law be enforced."[4]

The principle of individual criminal responsibility for violations of certain international norms has now been codified in treaty law. The Rome Statute of the International Criminal Court (ICC), (Rome Statute of the International Criminal Court, 2002), adopted in 1998, provides the most comprehensive codification to date of international criminal law. Included within its subject matter jurisdiction are the crimes of aggression,[5] genocide, war crimes, and crimes against humanity. The treaty has been widely ratified, and its Assembly of States Parties aspires to universal participation.

Notwithstanding the fact that these norms directly bind individual human beings, it is essential to bear in mind that these norms were generated in an interstate legal system. Thus, for example, certain crimes will require an interstate element in order to engage the criminal responsibility of the individual under international law.

---

4. International Military Tribunal (Nuremberg) 41 AJIL 172 (1947) at 221.

5. Although included in the Rome Statute, the crime of aggression was left undefined. The ICC cannot prosecute this crime until a definition is adopted by the Assembly of States Parties to the Rome Statute.

Overview of International Criminal Courts

Beginning with the creation of the post-World War II International Military Tribunals at Nuremberg and Tokyo, the international community has established a number of international criminal courts over the course of the past 60 years. In the early 1990s the UN Security Council established two *ad hoc* tribunals – the International Criminal Tribunals for the former Yugoslavia and Rwanda. In 1998, the ICC Statute was adopted, and that Court was legally established in 2002. Each of these courts applies international criminal law directly to the individual perpetrators being prosecuted.

In addition to these quintessentially international courts, a number of so-called hybrid, or internationalized courts have also been created, such as the Special Court for Sierra Leone and the Extraordinary Chambers in the Courts of Cambodia. These hybrid institutions, composed of national and international officials, apply international criminal law directly, or through the modality of domestic legislation.

WAR CRIMES

The Regulation of Armed Conflict under International Law

The traditional function of public international law is to regulate relations between and among states. This function continues even when these relations degenerate into armed conflict, for during such conflicts "[t]he right of belligerents to adopt means of injuring the enemy is not unlimited."[6]

The law of armed conflict, known also as the law of war, the *jus in bello*, or international humanitarian law (IHL), is one of the oldest subject areas of international law. It refers to the corpus of international norms that regulates the conduct of hostilities, and that provides protection for persons not taking part, or no longer taking part, in hostilities.

While it shares with international human rights law the purpose of protecting individuals, the two bodies of international law may be distinguished on several grounds. Most significantly, human rights law is primarily concerned with the way a state treats those under its jurisdiction,

---

6. Art. 22, Fourth Hague Convention of 1907.

while "[h]umanitarian law aims at placing restraints on the conduct of warfare so as to diminish its effects on the victims of the hostilities."[7] Humanitarian law must also be distinguished from the *jus ad bellum*, which regulates the lawfulness of a state's initial recourse to the use of armed force. Once an armed conflict has begun, the *jus ad bellum* gives way to the *jus in bello*.

Humanitarian law applies only in times of armed conflict or occupation. One of the strengths of IHL is that it applies on the facts, and is unconcerned with political labels. Thus, a formal declaration of war is not necessary to trigger the application of IHL so long as an armed conflict or occupation in fact exists.

The Evolution of International Humanitarian Law

The corpus of IHL rests on a set of fundamental principles, which at the same time constitute the earliest antecedents of modern humanitarian law.[8] These include the complementary principles of necessity and humanity, and of distinction and proportionality.

While the principle of humanity was aimed at reducing human suffering, it is tempered by the principle of military necessity, which reflects the interests of the warring parties in avoiding conferral of a military advantage on the opposing party to the conflict. Thus, traditional weapons were prohibited only if they caused *unnecessary* suffering.

A balance is similarly struck between the principle of distinction and the permissibility of civilian casualties in the form of proportionate collateral damage. The principle of distinction requires that "the Parties to the conflict shall at all times distinguish between the civilian population and combatants and between civilian objects and military objectives and accordingly shall direct their operations only against military objectives."[9] Civilian casualties may result, however, in the course of an

---

7. Prosecutor v. Dragoljub Kunarac, Radomir Kovac and Zoran Vukovic, IT- 96-23/1, Judgment, 470(i) (Trial Chamber II, February 22, 2001). Other distinctions between human rights and humanitarian law include the subjects of obligations, the institutions competent to determine violations, the period of application, the range of rights protected, and the sources of obligations.

8. These principles are historically rooted in moral philosophy. The doctrine of collateral damage, for example, follows from the Thomist doctrine of "double-effect."

9. Protocol Additional to the Geneva Conventions of 12 August 1949, and Relating to the Protection of Victims of International Armed Conflicts, (Protocol I) art. 48, 8 June 1977, 1125 UNTS 3 [hereinafter Additional Protocol I].

attack against a military objective. The lawfulness of such an attack will be preserved so long as the expected loss of civilian life is not "excessive in relation to the concrete and direct military advantage anticipated."[10]

As may be gleaned from these principles, many provisions of IHL are premised on a bargaining of sorts. For example, certain protected objects retain their protected status only so long as they are not used for purposes related to the hostilities. Thus, when fighters take shelter in a church, the church becomes a lawful military objective, losing the protection otherwise afforded to it under humanitarian law.[11]

The Combatants' Privilege

One of the fundamental rules of IHL is embodied in the "combatants' privilege." While the above-mentioned principles imposed restraints on the conduct of hostilities, the combatants' privilege affords lawful combatants a privilege to kill enemy combatants. Thus, while IHL regulates the means by which such killing is effected, lawful combatants are immunized from prosecution for the act of killing itself, so long as the principle of distinction was not violated.

Hague Law and Geneva Law

The nineteenth century saw the conclusion of the first multilateral treaties codifying the law of armed conflict. The most comprehensive codifications were the Hague Conventions of 1899 and 1907 and the Geneva Conventions of 1949, supplemented by the Additional Protocols of 1977. In general, these treaties track two different strands of humanitarian law, known simply as the Hague law and the Geneva law.

The Hague law consists primarily of restraints on the conduct of hostilities, including the outright prohibition of certain methods and means of warfare. The rules of the Hague law prohibit, for example, attacks against particular targets, such as undefended towns or religious institutions, and the employment of certain types of weapons, in particular those calculated to cause unnecessary suffering.

---

10. *Id.* art. 57.

11. Note, however, that if there were civilians in the church as well, the principle of proportionality would still apply. If the number of civilians present in the church vastly outnumbered the number of combatants, it is likely that the principle of proportionality would bar attacking the church in a manner that would result in the deaths of those civilians.

The Geneva law focuses on the protection of individuals who are not or are no longer taking part in hostilities. Each of the four Geneva Conventions protects a different category of such individuals. The First and Second Geneva Conventions protect sick and wounded soldiers in the field and at sea, respectively. The Third Convention regulates the treatment of prisoners of war. The protection of civilians is the exclusive province of the Fourth Convention. The Additional Protocols to the Geneva Conventions simultaneously update and merge the Hague and Geneva law.

Among the most basic rules of IHL, in addition to the principles noted above, are the following. Persons *hors de combat* (i.e., an individual who has been removed from combat, e.g., through sickness or detention) and those not taking direct part in hostilities must be protected and treated humanely without adverse discrimination. It is forbidden to kill or injure an enemy who surrenders or is *hors de combat*. The wounded and sick must be collected and cared for by the party that has them in its power. The Red Cross emblem, which is used to protect humanitarian or medical establishments and personnel, must be respected. Captured combatants and civilians under the authority of an adverse party are entitled to have their basic rights respected; in particular they must be protected against violence. All persons are entitled to basic judicial guarantees. Parties to the conflict cannot use weapons or methods of warfare causing unnecessary suffering. In addition, certain acts are specifically prohibited. These include torture, the taking of hostages, the use of human shields, rape, the imposition of collective penalties, pillage,[12] and reprisals[13] against protected[14] persons.

The Grave Breaches

The Geneva Conventions also establish a special penal regime for certain violations – the so-called "grave breaches." When a grave breach

---

12. Pillage is essentially theft of civilian property. It must be distinguished from the lawful act of requisitioning supplies needed by an occupying army.
13. A reprisal is an otherwise unlawful act committed in response to an unlawful act by the opposing party. Reprisals are employed to induce compliance by the opposing party.
14. As noted above, the scope of protection afforded by the Geneva Conventions is limited to certain groups of individuals. The bulk of the protection afforded under the Fourth Convention is limited to a particular group of civilians – "those who, at a given moment and in any manner whatsoever, find themselves, in case of a conflict or occupation, in the hands of a Party to the conflict or Occupying Power of which they are not nationals." *See* Geneva Convention relative to the Protection of Civilian Persons in Time of War (4th Geneva Convention), 75 U.N.T.S. 287, art. 4 (1949).

is committed, all States Parties are obliged to criminalize such conduct under their domestic law, to seek out the perpetrators, and to bring them to justice through prosecution or extradition.[15]

The Continuing Relevance of Customary Law

Notwithstanding the codification of humanitarian law, the general principles and customary law of war as developed through the centuries continue to apply in a residual manner, filling any gaps between the express provisions of treaty law. As set forth in the famous Martens clause (Meron, 2000):[16]

> Until a more complete code of the laws of war has been issued, the High Contracting Parties deem it expedient to declare that, in cases not included in the Regulations adopted by them, the inhabitants and the belligerents remain under the protection and the rule of the principles of the law of nations, as they result from the usages established among civilized peoples, from the laws of humanity, and the dictates of the public conscience.[17]

The existence of customary international law is particularly important because a number of states, including the United States, have failed to ratify the Additional Protocols to the 1949 Geneva Conventions. While these states would not be bound by those instruments as such, they would be bound by the rules contained therein to the extent that these rules had evolved into customary law.

---

15. *See* Geneva Convention for the Amelioration of the Condition of the Wounded and Sick in Armed Forces in the Field (1st Geneva Convention), 75 U.N.T.S. 31, art. 50 (1949) ("Grave breaches to which the preceding Article relates shall be those involving any of the following acts, if committed against persons or property protected by the Convention: willful killing, torture or inhuman treatment, including biological experiments, willfully causing great suffering or serious injury to body or health, and extensive destruction and appropriation of property, not justified by military necessity and carried out unlawfully and wantonly").

16. The "Martens clause," as it has come to be known, was included in the preamble of the Hague Conventions at the behest of F. F. de Martens, prominent jurist and Russian delegate to the 1899 Hague Peace Conference. The clause essentially invoked natural law to provide residual protection to victims of inhumane acts that were not expressly prohibited by the Convention. This clause also provided the foundation for the evolution of Crimes Against Humanity as they are understood today. *See* Theodor Meron, *The Martens Clause, Principles of Humanity, and Dictates of Public Conscience*, 94 AM. J. INT'L L. 78, 79 (2000). The International Court of Justice has found the Clause itself to constitute a rule of customary international law. Legality of the Threat or Use of Nuclear Weapons, 1996 I.C.J. 226, 257 (July 8).

17. Hague Conventions of 1907, preamble.

The Law of Non-International Armed Conflict

A more critical distinction than that between the Hague law and the Geneva law is the distinction between the law of international armed conflict and the law of non-international armed conflict.

Embedded in the classical system of international law, a system resting on the sovereign equality of states[18] and the related principle of non-intervention,[19] IHL is predominantly concerned with international (i.e., interstate) armed conflict. Among the four Geneva Conventions, only "Common Article 3" expressly applies to non-international armed conflict. Common Article 3 provides protection from only the most serious abuses.[20] While Protocol II also applies to non-international armed conflict, it provides significantly less protection to individuals than does Protocol I, which is applicable only in international armed conflict or occupation. Application of the Hague Conventions is similarly limited to situations of international armed conflict.[21]

While neither The Hague Conventions nor the Geneva Conventions define the phrase "armed conflict," definitions for both international and non-international armed conflict have been set forth in international jurisprudence. According to the jurisprudence of one international criminal court, an armed conflict exists "whenever there is a resort to armed force between States or protracted armed violence between governmental authorities and organized armed groups or between such groups within a State."[22]

A peculiar feature of the law of non-international armed conflict is its application to non-state groups. As noted above, the traditional subject

---

18. UN CHARTER, art. 2(1).

19. UN CHARTER, art. 2(7).

20. Common Article 3 prohibits the following acts against persons taking no active part in the hostilities: "[v]iolence to life and person, in particular murder of all kinds, mutilation, cruel treatment and torture; [the] [t]aking of hostages; [o]utrages upon personal dignity, in particular, humiliating and degrading treatment; [and] [t]he passing of sentences and the carrying out of executions without previous judgment pronounced by a regularly constituted court, affording all the judicial guarantees which are recognized as indispensable by civilized peoples."

21. Note, however, that the International Criminal Tribunal for the former Yugoslavia has greatly expanded the scope of norms applicable in non-international armed conflict. In the *Tadic* case, the Appeals Chamber found that certain norms of international armed conflict have evolved through customary law and now apply during non-international armed conflict as well. *Prosecutor v. Dusko Tadic*, IT-94-1-AR72, Decision on the Defense Motion for Interlocutory Appeal on Jurisdiction, 69 (October 2, 1995).

22. *Id.* at 70.

of international law is the state. However, over the course of the past century, the principle that only states could be the subjects of international legal obligations yielded to the changing values and nature of the international community. By its terms, Common Article 3 of the Geneva Conventions binds both states and non-state parties to non-international conflicts. In addition, certain norms of IHL have evolved into norms of international criminal law, which directly binds individuals.

The Law of Occupation

As noted above, IHL applies in times of occupation, as well as armed conflict. Indeed, the Geneva Conventions make clear that they apply to all cases of partial or total occupation, "even if the said occupation meets with no armed resistance."

According to the Fourth Hague Convention of 1907, "Territory is considered occupied when it is actually placed under the authority of the hostile army." However, jurisprudence suggests that the term "occupation," as used in the Fourth Geneva Convention (Civilians), has a broader meaning. According to the Trial Chamber of the International Criminal Tribunal for the former Yugoslavia (ICTY) in the *Naletilic* case, "the application of the law of occupation as it effects 'individuals' as civilians protected under Geneva Convention IV does not require that the occupying power have actual authority. For the purposes of those individuals' rights, a state of occupation exists upon their falling into 'the hands of the occupying power.'"

War Crimes as Crimes under International Law

As noted in the Introduction, it was the establishment of the International Military Tribunals[23] in the aftermath of World War II that consolidated the principle of individual criminal responsibility and spurred the development of international criminal law.[24] Thus, the overwhelming

---

23. At the close of World War II, the Allies established the International Military Tribunal at Nuremberg as well as the International Military Tribunal for the Far East. While the former was established on the basis of a multilateral treaty, the latter was created on the basis of a unilateral order by the Supreme Commander of the Allied Powers.

24. As noted above, although international criminal law can refer to various distinct bodies of international law, ranging from extradition treaties to mutual assistance agreements, in this chapter it is used to refer to that body of international norms the breach of which gives rise to the criminal responsibility of the individual under international law.

majority of international crimes that were given cognizance by the international community at that time were those relating to war; i.e., violations of humanitarian law. In addition, the commission of international crimes, by their very nature and scale, will often coincide with times of massive upheaval, such as that which occurs during periods of armed conflict.

"War crimes" are essentially criminal violations of IHL (i.e., violations of those norms of IHL which are deemed to give rise to individual criminal responsibility). Genocide and crimes against humanity are distinct from war crimes in that they need not be committed in times of armed conflict. Nonetheless, war crimes comprise the richest array of norms within the Rome Statute (Rome Statute of the International Criminal Court, 2002).

It must be noted, however, that not all violations of IHL will constitute war crimes. The breach of some norms will give rise only to state responsibility (the traditional form of responsibility in international law), and not the responsibility of the individual perpetrator. When the drafters of the ICTY Statute began to develop the subject matter jurisdiction of the Tribunal, they were faced with the challenge of determining which violations of IHL gave rise to individual criminal responsibility. The first category of war crimes they included in the Statute was the category of "grave breaches" as set forth in the 1949 Geneva Conventions. Because such breaches were the subject of a mandatory penal regime in the Conventions, the drafters of those Conventions had clearly intended that the breach of such norms should give rise to criminal responsibility. The other category of war crimes included in the ICTY Statute referred simply to the "laws and customs of war," essentially leaving to the judges the question of which violations of IHL would constitute war crimes.

Thus, in the *Tadic* decision, the Appeals Chamber developed a framework for analyzing which norms of IHL gave rise to individual criminal responsibility, and could thus be prosecuted before the Tribunal. The primary criteria set forth were the character of the norm itself, the severity of the violation, and the interest of the international community in its repression.[25]

Further, for an act to constitute a war crime, a nexus must be established between the alleged offence and the armed conflict which gives rise to the applicability of international humanitarian law. The *ad hoc* tribunals have determined that such a nexus exists where an act is

---

25. *Tadic* Appeal Decision, 128.

closely related to an armed conflict; i.e., if the act was committed in furtherance of an armed conflict, or under the guise of an armed conflict. They have cited as factors in this determination: the fact that the perpetrator is a combatant; the fact that the victim is a member of the opposing party; the fact that the act may be said to serve the ultimate goal of a military campaign; and the fact that the crime is committed as part of, or in the context, of the perpetrator's official duties.

Unlike crimes against humanity, war crimes need not be committed as part of a broader pattern of crimes. A single act may constitute a war crime so long as it is somehow connected to an armed conflict. However, the ICC Statute stipulates that the "Court shall have jurisdiction in respect of war crimes in particular when committed as part of a plan or policy or as part of a large-scale commission of such crimes."[26]

The enumeration of war crimes in the Rome Statute is the most extensive to date, and is widely regarded as a progressive development of the law, as opposed to a codification of customary law existing at the time of its adoption. This poses no problem for the ICC since its jurisdiction is prospective. The fact that the Rome Statute criminalizes the conduct is sufficient to render the conduct prosecutable by the ICC. Nonetheless, many of the crimes included in the Statute were already recognized under customary law.

CRIMES AGAINST HUMANITY

The notion of crimes against humanity is derived in part from natural law, and is linked to the above-mentioned Martens Clause. These crimes were first prosecuted at Nuremberg and were included in the subject matter jurisdiction of all subsequent international criminal courts.

The Rome Statute provides a modern definition of crimes against humanity. Broadly speaking, the definition can be divided into the *chapeau*, or contextual elements of crimes against humanity, and the enumerated acts.

Article 7(1) of the Rome Statute reads:

> For the purpose of this Statute, "crime against humanity" means any of the following acts when committed as part of a widespread or systematic attack directed against any civilian population, with knowledge of the attack.

---

26. ICC Statute, art. 8.

a. Murder;
b. Extermination;
c. Enslavement;
d. Deportation or forcible transfer of population;
e. Imprisonment or other severe deprivation of physical liberty in violation of fundamental rules of international law;
f. Torture;
g. Rape, sexual slavery, enforced prostitution, forced pregnancy, enforced sterilization, or any other form of sexual violence of comparable gravity;
h. Persecution against any identifiable group or collectivity on political, racial, national, ethnic, cultural, religious, gender as defined in paragraph 3, or other grounds that are universally recognized as impermissible under international law, in connection with any act referred to in this paragraph or any crime within the jurisdiction of the Court;
i. Enforced disappearance of persons;
j. The crime of apartheid;
k. Other inhumane acts of a similar character intentionally causing great suffering, or serious injury to body or to mental or physical health.

Thus, crimes against humanity require that there be an act, committed as part of an overarching attack, of which the actor is aware.

Widespread or Systematic Attack

Definition of Attack

The definition of an attack is fairly nebulous, but may be generally defined as an unlawful act, event, or series of events. An "attack" does not necessarily require the use of armed force; it could involve other forms of inhumane mistreatment of the civilian population.[27]

---

27. *See* Prosecutor v. Laurent Semanza, ICTR-97-20, Judgment and Sentence, ¶ 327 (Trial Chamber III, May 15, 2003). *See also* Prosecutor v. Milomir Stakic, IT-97-24, Judgment, ¶ 623 (Trial Chamber II, July 31, 2003) (clarifying the difference between an attack and armed conflict: "an attack can precede, outlast, or continue during the armed conflict, but it need not be part of it and is not limited to the use of armed force; it encompasses any mistreatment of the civilian population").

Widespread or Systematic

The Rome Statute formulates the scale and organization criteria of an attack as disjunctive, allowing jurisdiction over attacks of either massive scale or based upon some degree of planning or organization.

While the Rome Statute defines neither "widespread" nor "systematic," delegations understood "widespread" to mean a "multiplicity of persons" or a "massive attack," and "systematic" to encompass a developed policy or a high degree of organization and planning of the acts. Under ICTY and ICTR jurisprudence, "widespread" has been interpreted to include both a large number of acts spread across time or geography, as well as a single or limited number of acts committed on a large scale.[28] For the ICTR, "systematic" generally refers to the organized or planned nature of the attack.[29] However, this planning can be done by any organization or group, rather than being limited to the State or military bodies.[30] The ICTY has similarly defined systematicity, and pointed to relevant factors in determining this element.[31] The relevant factors include:

- The existence of a policy, plan, or ideology on which the attack is perpetrated, that supports destruction, persecution, or a weakening of the targeted community;
- The perpetration of the attack on a very large scale against a group of civilians or the repeated and continuous commission of inhumane acts linked to one another;
- The use of significant public or private resources, whether military or other; and
- The involvement of high-level political and/or military authorities in the establishment and perpetration of the plan.

Policy Requirement

Under the Rome Statute, the attacks must meet two threshold requirements: the attack must be "widespread or systematic," and must

---

28. *See* Prosecutor v. Jean-Paul Akayesu, ICTR-96-4, Opinion and Judgment, ¶ 580 (Trial Chamber I, September 2, 1998); *Tadic* Trial Judgment, ¶ 648; Prosecutor v. Dragoljub Kunarac, Radomir Kovac and Zoran Vukovic, IT- 96-23/1, Judgment, ¶ 94 (Appeals Chamber, June 12, 2002).

29. *See Akayesu* Trial Judgment, 173.

30. Prosecutor v. Ignace Bagilishema, ICTR-95-1A-T, Judgment, ¶ 78 (Trial Chamber I, June 7, 2001).

31. Prosecutor v. Blaskic, IT-95-14, Judgment, ¶ 203 (Trial Chamber I, March 2, 2000).

consist of "a course of conduct involving the multiple commission of acts referred to in paragraph 1 against any civilian population, pursuant to or in furtherance of a State or organizational policy to commit such attack."[32]

Under earlier definitions of crimes against humanity, such as those found in the Statutes of the ICTY and ICTR, it was not necessary to prove the existence of a policy or plan to commit such crimes.[33] Nonetheless, evidence of such a plan or policy would be useful in proving the "widespread" or "systematic" nature of the attack.

Directed Against Any Civilian Population

Definition of Civilian Population

The ICTY and ICTR Statutes as well as jurisprudence state that the attack must be committed against *any* civilian population. This qualification has been interpreted to mean that the inclusion of non-civilians (military forces or those who have previously borne arms in a conflict) does not necessarily deprive the population of its civilian character.[34] However, the targeted population must remain predominantly civilian in nature.[35] Further, according to ICTR and ICTY jurisprudence, it is the situation of the victim at the time of the attack, and not the victim's status, that should be the focus of the inquiry.[36] Thus, in the context of crimes against humanity, a non-civilian may still be considered a civilian if at the time of the attack he or she was not participating in the hostilities.

The population requirement refers to the idea that enough people must be targeted to show that the attack was directed against "a population" as opposed to limited and randomly selected individuals.[37] However,

---

32. Rome Statute, arts. 7(1) and 7(2) (a).

33. *See Semanza* Trial Judgment, 326, 329; *Kunarac* Appeal Judgment, 89, 98.

34. *See Tadic* Trial Judgment, 638; *Blaskic* Trial Judgment, 209; Prosecutor v. Zoran Kupreskic, Mirjan Kupreskic, Vlatko Kupreskic, Drago Josipovic, Dragan Papic, Vladimir Santic, a/k/a "Vlado," IT-95-16, Judgment 568 (Trial Chamber II, January 14, 2000); *Akayesu* Trial Judgment, at n. 146.

35. *See Akayesu* Trial Judgment, 575 (citing Prosecutor v. Dragoljub Kunarac, Radomir Kovac and Zoran Vukovic, IT-95-13-R61, Rule 61 Decision of 3 April 1996 (Trial Chamber II, April 3, 1996)).

36. *See Bagilishema* Trial Judgment, 79 (citing *Blaskic* Trial Judgment, 214 ("[t]he specific situation of the victim at the moment of the crimes committed, rather than his status, must be taken into account in determining his standing as a civilian")).

37. *See Stakic* Trial Judgment, 624.

the ICTY has held that "population" need not be the entire population of a state, city, or town.[38]

Mens Rea

The *mens rea* element for crimes against humanity requires that the prosecution prove the actor's knowledge of, but not necessarily responsibility for, the overarching attack. It is the association with a widespread or systematic overarching attack that elevates these offenses to the status of violations against "humanity." Thus, to satisfy the *mens rea* element of crimes against humanity, the defendant must be aware of the attack that makes his or her act a crime against humanity.

In practice, this means that the perpetrator must have knowledge of the attack and some understanding of the relationship between his or her acts and the attack.[39] Under ICTY jurisprudence, knowingly running the risk that an act may be part of a greater attack is sufficient to establish the mens rea.[40] However, the Appeals Chamber in *Kunarac* made clear that the perpetrator need not know the details of the attack.[41] Similarly, the ICC Elements of Crimes affirms that knowledge of the attack does not necessitate complete knowledge of the detailed character of the attack or the plan or policy behind it.[42]

Both *ad hoc* tribunals note that motive is entirely separate.[43] The perpetrator need not share a purpose or policy goal behind the attack with any other entity.[44] Similarly, it is irrelevant whether the accused intended the acts to be directed against the targeted population or just the particular victim.[45]

---

38. *See Tadic* Trial Judgment, 644.

39. Prosecutor v. Clement Kayishema and Obed Ruzindana, ICTR-95-1-T, Judgment, 131-32 (Trial Chamber II, May 21, 1999) ("The perpetrator must knowingly commit crimes against humanity in the sense that he must understand the overall context of his act.").

40. *See Kunarac*, Appeal Judgment, 102.

41. *See id.*

42. Preparatory Commission for the International Criminal Court, Report of the Preparatory Commission for the International Criminal Court, Part II, Finalized draft text of the Elements of Crimes, Addendum, at 9, U.N. Doc. PCNICC/2000/1/Add.2 (2000) [hereinafter PrepCom Elements of Crimes].

43. *See Kunarac* Appeal Judgment, 103; *Kupreskic* Trial Judgment, 558. At most, evidence that the perpetrator committed the acts for purely personal reasons would be indicative of a rebuttable assumption that the perpetrator was not aware that his or her acts were part of that attack. *See Kunarac* Appeal Judgment, 103.

44. *See Kunarac* Appeal Judgment, 103.

45. *See id.*

The ICC Elements of Crimes expands upon the statutes of the *ad hoc* tribunals by including a provision that specifically provides for "first actors." "First actors" – initiators of the attack or offenders whose acts take place at the cusp of the attack – will supply the requisite *mens rea* if an intent to further the emerging attack is proved.[46]

No Discrimination Requirement

Although discriminatory grounds were necessary to establish crimes against humanity under the ICTR Statute,[47] an overwhelming majority at the Rome Conference opposed the inclusion of a discrimination requirement for crimes against humanity. Many delegations were concerned that the inclusion of discrimination as a contextual element could have led to a limiting construction of the provision that would have excluded jurisdiction over otherwise severe atrocities.[48] Accordingly, the *chapeau* in the Rome Statute does not contain a discrimination requirement. This interpretation is consistent with ICTY jurisprudence, which has affirmed that discrimination is not an element of crimes against humanity, except for persecution.[49]

Nexus between the Act and the Attack

Both the ICTR and ICTY have interpreted their own Statutes to require a nexus between the act and an attack.[50] Thus, crimes against humanity consist of individual "acts" that will fall under, be connected with, or exist during a larger "attack."[51]

---

46. PrepCom Elements of Crimes, at 9.

47. It should be noted that the ICTR has recognized that this discriminatory element is a jurisdictional requirement specific to the ICTR and not a reflection of customary international law. *See Akayesu* Trial Judgment, 175.

48. For instance, because discriminatory grounds are limited to enumerated discriminations (political, racial, etc.), an executed policy of extermination directed at victims not within those specifically prohibited classes would not have been justiciable.

49. Prosecutor v. Dusko Tadic a/k/a "Dule," IT-94-1-A, Judgment, 249 (Appeals Chamber, July 15, 1999). *See also* Prosecutor v. Dario Kordic and Mario Cerkez, IT-95-14/2, Judgment, 211 (Trial Chamber III, February 26, 2001).

50. *See Semanza* Trial Judgment, 330; *Tadic* Appeal Judgment, 251.

51. Each act within Article 3(a)-(i) has its own requirements, but each must be part of the greater attack required by the *chapeau*. The enumerated acts which may rise to the level of crimes against humanity are the same in the ICTR and ICTY statutes. Statute of the International Criminal Tribunal for the Former Yugoslavia, S.C. Res. 827, U.N. SCOR, 3217th mtg., art. 5, U.N. Doc. S/RES/827 (1993); ICTR Statute, art. 3.

ICTR jurisprudence has determined that the act does not need to be committed at the same time or place as the attack, or share the same features, but it must, on some essential level, form part of the attack.[52] It must share some relation, temporal or geographical, with the attack. To meet this requirement, the act does not necessarily have to be committed against the same population as the broader attack of which it is a part.[53]

No Armed Conflict Requirement

The nexus between an act and an attack must be distinguished from the question of whether the act must be "committed in armed conflict." While the Statute of the ICTY included this requirement as a jurisdictional element, no such element is required under customary international law.[54] Accordingly, the Rome Statute does not contain an armed conflict requirement, allowing prosecution of acts perpetrated during peacetime as well as both internal and international armed conflicts.

GENOCIDE[55]

Genocide, in General

The term "genocide" was coined by the Polish-American jurist Raphael Lemkin in the early 1940s to describe the intentional destruction of certain groups. Writing in the midst of the Holocaust, Lemkin's work was heavily influenced by the events of World War II (Lemkin, 1947).

---

52. *Semanza* Trial Judgment, 329 ("Although the act need not be committed at the same time and place as the attack or share all of the features of the attack, it must, by its characteristics, aims, nature, or consequence objectively form part of the discriminatory attack."). *Cf Tadic* Appeal Judgment 251.

53. *See Semanza* Trial Judgment 330. Although the act does not have to be committed against the same population, if it is committed against the same population, that characteristic may be used to demonstrate the nexus between the act and the attack.

54. *See Tadic* Appeal Judgment, 249. Although the ICTY Statute retains an armed conflict requirement for crimes against humanity, the *Tadic* Appeals Chamber explicitly recognized that this requirement is a jurisdictional element only and does not reflect customary international law. *Id.*

55. This section is based largely upon J. Cerone, "Recent Developments in the Law of Genocide" in S. Vardy & T. Tooley, *Ethnic Cleansing in 20th-Century Europe*, Columbia University Press, New York (2003).

Although the term "genocide" did not appear in the Nuremberg Charter or in the judgment of the International Military Tribunal at Nuremberg, its definition was set forth in the 1948 Genocide Convention, which states:

> "genocide" means any of the following acts committed with intent to destroy, in whole or in part, a national, ethnical, racial or religious group, as such:
>
> a. Killing members of the group;
> b. Causing serious bodily or mental harm to members of the group;
> c. Deliberately inflicting on the group conditions of life calculated to bring about its physical destruction in whole or in part;
> d. Imposing measures intended to prevent births within the group;
> e. Forcibly transferring children of the group to another group.

This definition is reiterated almost verbatim in all relevant international legal instruments. Broadly speaking, the definition can be divided into a mental element (the necessary intent to destroy the group as such) and a physical element (the commission of at least one of the enumerated acts).

Distinctive Features of the Definition

A few preliminary observations about the definition are important. First, genocide is a specific intent crime. This special intent requirement (or *dolus specialis*) is an element of the crime. The perpetrator must have the intent to destroy, in whole or in part, a group as such.

Second, killing is not expressly required. The perpetrator need only commit one of the enumerated acts with the required intent. However, the *travaux préparatoires* make clear that the definition of genocide set forth in the Convention was not intended to encompass "cultural genocide;" nor was it intended to provide protection for political groups (Kunz, 1949).

Third, unlike war crimes, the crime of genocide need not occur in the context of an armed conflict. Additionally, although both genocide and crimes against humanity can be committed in times of peace, these two crimes should also be distinguished from one another. As the ICTY Trial Chamber noted in the case of *Prosecutor v Kupreskic*, genocide is an extreme and most inhumane form of the crime against humanity of persecution; its *mens rea* requires proof of the intent not only to discriminate, but also to destroy, in whole or in part, the group to which the victims of the genocide belong.[56]

Finally, the prohibition of genocide has entered the corpus of customary international law. Thus, the obligation to prevent and punish genocide exists independently of a state's treaty obligations (i.e., even states not parties to the Convention are bound by this obligation).[57] Further, this norm has acquired the status of *jus cogens*, meaning that it is a higher-order norm overriding conflicting obligations and voiding conflicting treaties.[58]

Elaboration of the Definition through International Jurisprudence – The ICTs

The jurisprudence of the International Criminal Tribunals (ICTs) for the former Yugoslavia and Rwanda has contributed to the elaboration of the law of genocide, particularly as applied to individual perpetrators.

Individual Criminal Responsibility

Early on the ICTY confirmed that there is individual criminal responsibility under international law for the commission of genocide.[59] Thus, the commission of genocide can give rise to both state responsibility and individual criminal responsibility.

Elaboration of the Definition

The ICTR has adopted a fairly expansive interpretation of the definition of genocide; the ICTY less so. However, there is extensive cross-fertilization between the two tribunals, as each frequently cites cases of the other, leading to harmonization of their decisions.

---

56. Prosecutor v. Zoran Kupreskic, Mirjan Kupreskic, Vlatko Kupreskic, Drago Josipovic, Dragan Papic, Vladimir Santic, also known as "Vlado," IT-95-16, Judgment ¶ 636, (Trial Chamber II, January 14, 2000).

57. See *Reservations to the Convention on Genocide* (Advisory Opinion), ICJ Reports 1951.

58. Human Rights Committee, General Comment 6, 30 July 1982. See also *Case Concerning Application of the Convention on the Prevention and Punishment of the Crime of Genocide (Bosnia and Herzegovina v. Yugoslavia (Serbia and Montenegro))* (separate opinion of Judge Lauterpacht), 1993 I.C.J. 325. It should be noted, however, that the doctrine of *jus cogens* is not universally accepted.

59. The Prosecutor v. Dusko Tadic, IT-94-1-AR72, Decision on the Defense Motion for Interlocutory Appeal on Jurisdiction, at RP D6413-D6491 (October 2, 1995).

PROTECTED GROUPS. The ICTR has examined the nature of the groups listed in the definition and extracted what it deemed a common criterion – "that membership in such groups would seem to be normally not challengeable by its members, who belong to it automatically, by birth, in a continuous and often irremediable manner."[60] It determined that any permanent, stable group should be protected.

The ICTY took a similarly broad approach by holding that a group may be defined with reference to the perspective of the perpetrator. In the *Jelisic* case, the ICTY held:

> to attempt to define a national, ethnical or racial group today using objective and scientifically irreproachable criteria would be a perilous exercise whose result would not necessarily correspond to the perception of the persons concerned by such categorisation. Therefore, it is more appropriate to evaluate the status of a national, ethnical or racial group from the point of view of those persons who wish to single that group out from the rest of the community.[61]

The Tribunal stated further that a positive or negative approach could be used in making this determination.[62] A positive approach, as defined by the Tribunal, would involve distinguishing a group by characteristics which perpetrators deem particular to that group. A negative approach would be the case where perpetrators distinguish themselves as an ethnic, racial, religious, or national group distinct from the other group or groups.

Enumerated Acts

In the *Akayesu* case, the first genocide case prosecuted before an international criminal court, the ICTR elaborated upon the possible acts that constitute genocide when committed with the requisite intent.

KILLING MEMBERS OF THE GROUP. With regard to the first enumerated act – killing members of the group, the ICTR has employed a somewhat narrow interpretation by requiring that the killing amount to

---

60. *See* Prosecutor v. Jean-Paul Akayesu, ICTR-96-4, Opinion and Judgment 511 (Trial Chamber I, September 2, 1998).

61. Prosecutor v. Moran Jelisic, IT-95-10, Judgment ¶ 70 (Trial Chamber I, December 14, 1999).

62. *Jelisic*, Trial Chamber at 71. *But see* Prosecutor v. Milomir Stakic, IT-97-24, Judgment ¶ 732 (Trial Chamber II, July 31, 2003) (stating that "the Trial Chamber does not agree with the 'negative approach' taken by the Trial Chamber in *Jelisic*").

murder (a specific intent crime).[63] However, there is nothing particularly new in this holding, as killing with the intent to destroy the group will generally mean that the perpetrator intended to kill the victim in any case.

CAUSING SERIOUS BODILY OR MENTAL HARM TO MEMBERS OF THE GROUP. Regarding the second enumerated act, the ICTR stated, "Causing serious bodily or mental harm to members of the group does not necessarily mean that the harm is permanent and irremediable."[64] In doing so, it cited the *Eichmann* case for the proposition that "serious bodily or mental harm of members of the group can be caused 'by the enslavement, starvation, deportation and persecution [. . .] and by their detention in ghettos, transit camps and concentration camps in conditions which were designed to cause their degradation, deprivation of their rights as human beings, and to suppress them and cause them inhumane suffering and torture.'"[65] Ultimately, the ICTR took serious bodily or mental harm, "without limiting itself thereto, to mean acts of torture, be they bodily or mental, inhumane or degrading treatment, persecution."[66] The *Akayesu* Trial Chamber expressly found that sexual violence fell into this category, and ultimately pointed to acts of rape in this case as genocidal acts.

DELIBERATELY INFLICTING ON THE GROUP CONDITIONS OF LIFE CALCULATED TO BRING ABOUT ITS PHYSICAL DESTRUCTION IN WHOLE OR IN PART. The ICTR held that the means of deliberately inflicting on the group conditions of life calculated to bring about its physical destruction, in whole or part, "include, *inter alia*, subjecting a group of people to a subsistence diet, systematic expulsion from homes and the reduction of essential medical services below minimum requirement."[67]

IMPOSING MEASURES INTENDED TO PREVENT BIRTHS WITHIN THE GROUP. Within this category of measures, the ICTR included sexual mutilation, the practice of sterilization, forced birth control, separation of the sexes and prohibition of marriages.[68] In addition, it held that in a culture where membership in the group is determined by the identity of

---

63. *Akayesu*, Trial Chamber, at 501. Similarly, the ICTY has defined "killing" as an "intentional but not necessarily premeditated act[]." *Stakic*, Trial Chamber at 515.
64. *Akayesu*, Trial Chamber, at 502.
65. *Id.* at 503.
66. *Id.* at 504.
67. *Id.* at 506.
68. *Id.* at 507.

the father, deliberate impregnation during rape by a man not of the group[69] could also constitute such a measure. The Tribunal further determined that such measures could be psychological in nature. It stated, "For instance, rape can be a measure intended to prevent births when the person raped refuses subsequently to procreate, in the same way that members of a group can be led, through threats or trauma, not to procreate."[70]

FORCIBLY TRANSFERRING CHILDREN OF THE GROUP TO ANOTHER GROUP. In line with its expansive interpretation of the first four enumerated acts, the Tribunal opined that the objective of the fifth enumerated act "is not only to sanction a direct act of forcible physical transfer, but also to sanction acts of threats or trauma which would lead to the forcible transfer of children from one group to another."[71]

The Intent Requirement

In addition to the *mens rea* of the underlying crime, genocide requires proof of a *dolus specialis*; that is, a specific intent to commit genocide. For that reason, genocide is not easy to prove. Recognizing that the special intent inherent in the crime of genocide is a mental factor which is difficult, even impossible, to determine, the *Akayesu* Trial Chamber noted that "in the absence of a confession from the accused, his intent can be inferred from a certain number of presumptions of fact."[72]

In the *Akayesu* case, the ICTR considered that it was possible to infer the genocidal intent of a particular act from: (1) the general context of the perpetration of other culpable acts systematically directed against that same group, whether these acts were committed by the same offender or by others; (2) the scale of atrocities committed, their general nature, in a region or a country; and (3) the deliberate and systematic targeting of victims on account of their membership of a particular group, while excluding the members of other groups.[73]

---

69. *Id.* at 507 ("In patriarchal societies, where membership of a group is determined by the identity of the father, an example of a measure intended to prevent births within a group is the case where, during rape, a woman of the said group is deliberately impregnated by a man of another group, with the intent to have her give birth to a child who will consequently not belong to its mother's group").
70. *Id.* at 508.
71. *Id.* at 509.
72. *Id.* at 523.
73. *Id.* at 523.

The ICTY has held that the requisite intent may be inferred from "the perpetration of acts which violate, or which the perpetrators themselves consider to violate the very foundation of the group – acts which are not in themselves covered by the list in Article 4(2) but which are committed as part of the same pattern of conduct."[74] In that case, the ICTY found that "this intent derives from the combined effect of speeches or projects laying the groundwork for and justifying the acts, from the massive scale of their destructive effect and from their specific nature, which aims at undermining what is considered to be the foundation of the group."[75]

The ICT has provided additional examples of factors that can be used to infer genocidal intent. In the *Ruzindana* case, the Tribunal referred to a "pattern of purposeful action," which might include: (1) the physical targeting of the group or their property; (2) the use of derogatory language toward members of the targeted group; (3) the weapons employed and the extent of bodily injury; and (4) the methodical way of planning, the systematic manner of killing.[76]

"IN WHOLE OR IN PART." With respect to the "in whole or in part" dimension of the intended destruction, the ICTY affirmed the position of the International Law Commission that complete annihilation from every corner of globe is not required.[77] In particular, the *Jelisic* Tribunal held that the intent may extend only to a limited geographical area.[78] Although there is no numeric threshold of victims necessary to establish genocide, the ICTY held that "in part" means in *substantial* part. It further stated that a substantial part might include a large number or a representative faction. If the latter, that representative faction must be destroyed in such a way so as to threaten the survival of the group as a whole.[79]

---

74. *Id.* at 524.

75. *Id.*

76. Prosecutor v. Clement Kayishema and Obed Ruzindana, 1: ICTR-95-1; 2: ICTR-96-10, Judgment, ¶ 93 (Trial Chamber, May 21, 1999).

77. Prosecutor v. Moran Jelisic, IT-95-10, Judgment (Trial Chamber I, December 14, 1999).

78. *Accord Prosecutor v. Kristic*, IT- 98-33, Judgment, 590 (Trial Chamber I, Aug. 2, 2001) (noting that although the killing of all members of a part of a group in a particular geographic area may result in less killings than a campaign spread over a broad geographical area, it would "qualify as genocide if carried out with the intent to destroy the part of the group as such located in this small geographic area").

79. *See Jelisic*, Trial Chamber, 83 (Trial Chamber I, December 14, 1999). *See also* 18 USC 1093 (2000) ("'Substantial part' means a part of a group of such numerical significance that the destruction or loss of that part would cause the destruction of the group as a viable entity within the nation of which such group is a part").

ROLE OF THE INDIVIDUAL PERPETRATOR. The Tribunal in *Jelisic* also dealt with the issue of the role of the individual perpetrator in the commission of genocide. Generally, the tribunals have first determined whether genocide occurred in an area, and then proceeded to determine whether an individual has shared the genocidal intent. In *Jelisic*, the ICTY indicated that an individual could be deemed responsible for genocide where he was one of many executing an overall, higher level planned genocide, or where he individually committed genocide.[80] Thus, the Tribunal indicated that an individual alone could be guilty of committing genocide; however, of course, it is still very difficult to prove if the acts were not widespread and not backed by an organization or system.

GENOCIDE V. FORCED EXPULSION. It cannot be emphasized enough that the genocidal intent is determinative of whether the crime occurred. In this context, it is important to recall that although the *ad hoc* tribunals have held that forced expulsion may be one of the acts constituting genocide, this expulsion must be carried out with the intent to destroy the group if that act is to constitute genocide. Thus in the *Kupreskic* case, the ICTY found that:

> The primary purpose of the massacre was to expel the Muslims from the village, by killing many of them, by burning their houses, slaughtering their livestock, and by illegally detaining and deporting the survivors to another area. The ultimate goal of these acts was to spread terror among the population so as to deter the members of that particular ethnic group from ever returning to their homes.[81]

The Tribunal thus held that this was a case of the crime against humanity of persecution, and that it was not a case of genocide.[82]

Additional Element

The Elements of Crimes adopted for the ICC for each of the enumerated acts of genocide include a common element not explicitly required in prior instruments or in the jurisprudence of the ICTY or

---

80. *Jelisic*, Trial Chamber, 78.
81. *Kupreskic*, Trial Chamber at 749.
82. *Kupreskic*, Trial Chamber at 751 (But note that the Prosecutor agreed with the Tribunal in that case. Genocide was not charged). *Accord Stakic, supra* note 62, ¶ 519 ("A clear distinction must be drawn between physical destruction and mere dissolution of a group. The expulsion of a group or part of a group does not in itself suffice for genocide").

ICTR; namely, that the conduct must have taken place "in the context of a manifest pattern of similar conduct directed against that group or was conduct that could itself effect such destruction."

INDIVIDUAL CRIMINAL RESPONSIBILITY

International criminal law also governs the various modes of participation in international crimes. In an attempt to reach all guilty parties, international criminal law extends individual responsibility to all those who participate in international crimes, whether directly or indirectly. Thus, in addition to those who have directly committed the impugned act, international criminal law creates responsibility for all those who have planned, instigated, ordered, or otherwise aided and abetted in the planning, preparation or execution of a crime.[83] It also recognizes the responsibility of superiors where a superior fails to prevent or respond to criminal conduct by a subordinate.[84]

The mode of responsibility that forms the basis of an individual's criminal liability will also have implications for investigations. Two modes of responsibility of special relevance to this issue are joint criminal enterprise and command (or superior) responsibility.

Joint Criminal Enterprise

Joint criminal enterprise liability "entails individual responsibility for participation in a joint criminal enterprise to commit a crime."[85] According to the Appeals Chamber in *Tadic*, for joint criminal enterprise liability, three specific elements must be proved.

1. *A plurality of persons.* They need not be organized in a military, political or administrative structure.
2. *The existence of a common plan, design or purpose which amounts to or involves the commission of a crime provided for in the Statute.* There is no necessity for this plan, design or purpose to have been previously

---

83. Statute of the International Criminal Tribunal for the former Yugoslavia, S.C. Res. 827, U.N. SCOR, 3217th mtg., art. 7, U.N. Doc. S/RES/827 (1993) [hereinafter ICTY Statute]; Statute of the International Criminal Tribunal for Rwanda, S.C. Res. 955, U.N. SCOR, 49th Sess., 3453d mtg., Annex, art. 6(1), U.N. Doc. S/RES/955 (1994) [hereinafter ICTR Statute].
84. *Id.*
85. *Krstic* Trial Judgment, 480.

arranged or formulated. The common plan or purpose may materialise extemporaneously and be inferred from the fact that a plurality of persons acts in unison to put into effect a joint criminal enterprise.

3. *Participation of the accused in the common design* involving the perpetration of one of the crimes provided for in the Statute. This participation need not involve commission of a specific crime under one of those provisions (for example, murder, extermination, torture, rape, etc.), but may take the form of assistance in, or contribution to, the execution of the common plan or purpose.[86]

The requisite *mens rea* differs depending on whether the alleged crime:

a. was within the object of the joint criminal enterprise, or
b. went beyond the object of that enterprise, but was nevertheless a natural and foreseeable consequence of that enterprise."[87]

For the first type, where the crime is one that was an intended outcome of the joint criminal enterprise, "the prosecution must establish that the accused shared with the person who personally perpetrated the crime the state of mind required for that crime."[88] In the second set of circumstances, where a crime occurs that was not part of the original plan, responsibility for one or many other additional crimes may still be possible if the following two elements are met:

1. it was *foreseeable* that such a crime might be perpetrated by one or other members of the group and
2. the accused willingly took that risk.[89]

Responsibility of Commanders and Other Superiors

According to the ICTY Statute, a superior is responsible if he or she knew or had reason to know that a subordinate was about to commit a crime or had done so, and the superior failed to take the necessary and reasonable measures to prevent such acts or to punish the perpetrators thereof.

---

86. *Tadic* Appeal Judgment, 227; *see also Krstic* Trial Judgment, 490.
87. *Krstic* Trial Judgment, 492.
88. *Id.*
89. *Tadic* Appeal Judgment, 228 (emphasis in original).

That the commander/superior knew or had reason to know of the acts informs whether he or she is responsible for not preventing or punishing the perpetration of the crimes. It is this omission or negative action that elevates the responsibility of a commanding officer or superior to this level. Command or superior responsibility is therefore not a form of strict liability, but a type of imputed responsibility.[90] As the *Kordic* Trial Chamber explains:

> The type of responsibility provided for in Article 7(3) may be described as "indirect" as it does not stem from a "direct" involvement by the superior in the commission of a crime but rather from his omission to prevent or punish such offence, i.e., of his failure to act in spite of knowledge. This responsibility arises only where the superior is under a legal obligation to act.[91]

This element of responsibility arises from treaty law and customary international law, including Additional Protocol I to the Geneva Conventions establishing an affirmative duty for commanders to prevent and punish violations of international humanitarian law.[92] However, "only feasible measures in the power of a superior are required."[93]

The *Mucic* Trial Chamber developed three elements to determine whether command responsibility existed:

1. the existence of a superior-subordinate relationship;
2. the superior knew or had reason to know that the criminal act was about to be or had been committed; and
3. the superior failed to take the necessary and reasonable measures to prevent the criminal act or punish the perpetrator thereof.[94]

The *Naletilic* Trial Chamber also emphasized the importance of effective control in determining whether command responsibility arises.[95] Although actual knowledge cannot be presumed, the fact that an individual was a commanding officer may be used as an *indicium* of knowledge regarding the acts of his or her subordinates.[96] For a commander/superior to "have reason to know," ICTY jurisprudence dictates that:

---

90. *See Kordic* Trial Judgment, 365.
91. *Id.*
92. *See id.*
93. *Naletilic* Trial Judgment, 77.
94. Prosecutor v. Mucic, IT-96-21, Judgment, 346 (Trial Chamber II, November 16, 1998).
95. *See Naletilic* Trial Judgment, 66.
96. *See id.* 71.

a superior can be held criminally responsible only if some specific information was in fact available to him which would provide notice of offences committed by his subordinates. This information need not be such that it by itself was sufficient to compel the conclusion of the existence of such crimes. It is sufficient that the superior was put on further inquiry by the information, or, in other words, that it indicated the need for additional investigation in order to ascertain whether offences were being committed or about to be committed by his subordinates.[97]

IMPLICATIONS FOR INVESTIGATIONS

In many respects, the elements required for the various crimes identified above, as well as the modes of participation in these crimes, will present special challenges for investigation. The following examples will serve to illustrate this point.

For war crimes, prosecutors will first have to produce evidence that a state of armed conflict or occupation existed at the relevant time. To do so, they will have to establish that there has been a resort to armed force between States or protracted armed violence between governmental authorities and organized armed groups or between such groups within a State. Alternatively, they would have to demonstrate a state of occupation; i.e., that the relevant territory was actually placed under the authority of a hostile army.

They will also have to be able to demonstrate a nexus between the particular crime and that armed conflict or occupation. Thus, it is essential to uncover evidence that the perpetrator is a combatant, that the victim is a member of the opposing party, that the act may be said to serve the ultimate goal of a military campaign, or that the crime is committed as part of or in the context of the perpetrator's official duties.

In order to make out a case for crimes against humanity, prosecutors will have to show that there was a widespread or systematic attack directed against a civilian population, and that there was a nexus between the particular crime and that attack. As noted above, this could involve producing evidence of a policy, plan, or ideology on which the attack is perpetrated, that supports destruction, persecution, or a weakening of the targeted community; of the perpetration of the attack on a very large scale against a group of civilians or the repeated and continuous

---

97. *Id.* 74 (citing *Mucic* Trial Judgment, 393).

commission of inhumane acts linked to one another; of the use of significant public or private resources, whether military or other; or of the involvement of high-level political and/or military authorities in the establishment and perpetration of the plan.

For genocide, the primary hurdle for the prosecution will be the establishment of genocidal intent. In order for the relevant court to infer such intent, the prosecutors would have to produce evidence of a general context of the perpetration of other culpable acts systematically directed against that same group; of the deliberate and systematic targeting of victims on account of their membership of a particular group, while excluding the members of other groups; of the use of derogatory language toward members of the targeted group; of the weapons employed and the extent of bodily injury; or of methodical planning and the systematic manner of killing.

Finally, the establishment of joint criminal enterprise or superior responsibility requires proof of elements uncommon to ordinary criminal investigations. For joint criminal enterprise liability, the prosecution would have to establish the existence of a common plan, design or purpose which amounts to or involves the commission of an international crime, raising evidentiary challenges similar to those for proving the systematicity element of crimes against humanity.

As for superior responsibility, simply establishing a superior-subordinate relationship can be extremely complex in cases where this relationship exists *de facto*, but not *de jure*. Other evidentiary challenges arise in proving that a superior had access to information about atrocities committed in a distant battlefield.

All of these evidentiary challenges are in addition to those inherent in any criminal investigation, and they are magnified by the physical environments in which the crimes take place. Notwithstanding the difficulties encountered by the investigators of World War II atrocities, their task was simplified by the fact that the allies had police power throughout Germany after the war ended. This is not the case for today's international criminal courts. For several years after the establishment of the Yugoslav Tribunal, investigators and prosecutors had little or no access to the crime scenes, due to ongoing hostilities or lack of cooperation from local authorities. As this chapter is being written, prosecutors and investigators at the International Criminal Court have been unable to gain access to Darfur more than 18 months after the U.N. Security Council referred the situation there to the Court.

Any international criminal investigation must take into account this combination of legal, political, and logistical factors. A thorough understanding of international criminal law assists in the appreciation of their interaction.

REFERENCES

Kunz, J.L. (1949). The UN convention on genocide. *Amer. J. International Law, (43)*: 4.

Lemkin, R. (1947). Genocide as a crime under international law. *Amer. J. Internacional Law, (41)*:145.

Meron, T. (2000). The Martens clause, principles of humanity, and dictates of public conscience. *Am. J. International Law, (94)*: 78–79.

Rome Statute of the International Criminal Court (2002). http://www.un.org/law/icc/statute/english/rome_statute(e).pdf. Accessed on September 25th, 2006.

Chapter 3

INTERNATIONAL FORENSIC INVESTIGATIONS: LEGAL FRAMEWORK, ORGANISATION, AND PERFORMANCE

Juha Rainio, Kaisa Lalu and Antti Sajantila

INTRODUCTION

This chapter describes the legal framework of a forensic investigation of alleged human rights violations, the forensic team's assembling and logistics, security during the mission, and working standards. The descriptions are based mainly on the experiences of Finnish forensic experts in the former Yugoslavia. These experts performed investigations of human remains in the territory of the Republika Srpska in Bosnia and Herzegovina (BiH) under the mandate of the United Nations (UN Forensic Expert Team, UN-FET) in July 1996 (Ranta and Penttilä, 1999; Rainio et al., 2001a; Rainio, 2002), and then under the mandate of the European Union (EU-FET) in Kosovo, the Federal Republic of Yugoslavia (FRY), in December 1998 and January 1999 (Rainio et al., 2001a; Rainio et al., 2001b; Rainio et al., 2001c; Rainio et al., 2001d; Rainio, 2002). Moreover, Finnish forensic experts participated in international forensic investigations in Bosnia and Herzegovina conducted by the United Nations as well as in forensic investigations with many international teams in Kosovo in 1999 and 2000, supervised by the International Criminal Tribunal for the former Yugoslavia (ICTY) (Rainio, 2002). Table 3-1 displays schematically the procedures taken by an international forensic expert team during a mission.

TABLE 3-1. SCHEMATIC PRESENTATION OF PHASES IN
AN INTERNATIONAL FORENSIC MISSION

Request	Team Formation	Advance Preparations	Exhumation
Governments Intergovernmental organisations Non-governmental organisations Victims' relatives	Forensic pathologists Forensic anthropologists Forensic geneticists Forensic odontologists Forensic archaeologists Forensic investigators Other experts Technicians, secretaries	Mandate Tasks Equipment Working instructions Health issues Leaves of absence Insurance	Equipment Site security Chain of custody
Transportation	Autopsy	Documentation	Reporting
Individual resistant body bags Chain of custody	Equipment Model protocol Chain of custody Samples	Autopsy report X-rays Photographs Videos Laboratory results	Commissioner Team Public Media

The history of mankind contains numerous incidents of political or ethnic violence. In the twentieth century, however, the scale of such incidents and, particularly, public knowledge of these reached previously unknown dimensions (Rainio, 2002; Ferllini, 2003). Until the Second World War, no attempts had been made to construct a legal framework through which the international community could deal with cases of mass extermination (Blewitt, 1997). In addition, participation of forensic scientists in investigations of political or ethnic mass violence before the Second World War had been reported only exceptionally.

Subsequent investigations of victims of political or ethnic violence have more often involved forensic scientists. The medical scientific literature concerning forensic investigations in such instances has nevertheless been relatively sparse (Petersen and Vedel, 1994; Haglund, 2002; Rainio, 2002). Sometimes the data cannot be published for investigative reasons. On the other hand, in many publications the focus is not on the findings of the investigation (Rainio, 2002). Thus, even if forensic investigations have been conducted, investigative details, such as identification and number of the victims and their cause and manner of death, have not always been described. These aspects are, however, increasingly more often being published.

Forensic investigations of victims of alleged political mass violence are reported to have been performed, for example, in several countries of Latin America (Snow et al., 1984; Stover, 1985; Thomsen et al., 1989; Kirschner and Hannibal, 1994; Boles et al., 1995; Macilwain, 1995; Skolnick, 1995; Cordner and Ranson, 1997; Vanezis, 1997; Vanezis, 1999). Furthermore, the International Criminal Tribunal for Rwanda was appointed by the UN in November, 1994 after 500,000 to 800,000 people were claimed to have been killed from April to July 1994 (Dillner, 1994; Cordner and Ranson, 1997; Vanezis, 1999; Woodhouse, 1999).

Since 1992, the international community has been involved in investigating various armed conflicts that have arisen in the area of the former Yugoslavia. An International Criminal Tribunal for the former Yugoslavia (ICTY) was established in May 1993 by the UN Security Council (United Nations, 1995; Blewitt 1997; Cordner and Ranson, 1997; Cordner and McKelvie, 1998), and the Tribunal has, thereafter, issued several indictments for violations of international humanitarian law (Geiger, 1996). The forensic investigations of the victims have been performed by local forensic services (Marcikić et al., 1993; Kuzman et al., 1993) and by national and international forensic teams (Stanković, 1992; Zečević et al., 1993; Gunby, 1994; Strinovic, 1994; Primorac et al., 1996; Brkic et al., 1997; Chandrasiri, 1997; Brkic et al., 2000; Eriksson et al., 2000; Holck, 2000; Jacobs et al., 2000; Jacobs et al., 2001; Lorin de la Grandmaison and Durigon, 2001; Sprogøe-Jakobsen et al., 2001).

GENERAL BACKGROUND

The legal and moral basis underlying forensic investigation of situations in which extralegal, arbitrary or summary executions, torture or other violations of human rights are suspected is expressed in such international human rights standards as resolutions of the UN General Assembly, documents of the UN Economic and Social Council, the UN Commission on Human Rights, the UN Human Rights Committee, the UN Committee against Torture, the UN Committee on Crime Prevention and Control, and the UN congresses on the prevention of crime and the treatment of offenders (United Nations, 1957; United Nations, 1984a; United Nations, 1984b; United Nations, 1989).

According to a resolution of the UN Economic and Social Council (1989/65) (United Nations, 1989), governments shall prohibit by law all extralegal, arbitrary or summary executions in order to protect the right to life. Furthermore, states are obliged under international law to carry out impartial and exhaustive investigations into all allegations of massacres and other extrajudicial, summary or arbitrary killings, with a view to clarifying the circumstances, identifying those responsible, bringing them to justice, compensating the victims or their families, and taking all necessary actions to prevent the recurrence of similar acts in the future. The purpose of the investigation of all suspected cases shall also be to determine the cause, manner and time of death and to identify the body. The results of such investigations must be made public (United Nations, 1989).

Forensic investigations in cases of alleged political or ethnic violence can have various functions, principal of which are identification of victims, determination of their cause and manner of death and clarification of the circumstances surrounding death.

The identification of victims has several considerations, such as humanitarian and legal statistical aspects (van den Bos, 1980; Snow et al., 1984; Hill et al., 1988; Knight, 1991; Ludes et al., 1994; Stanković et al., 1994; Primorac et al., 1996; Kahana et al., 1997; Rainio, 2002). Official confirmation of victims' identity, according to local legislation as well as delivery of victims to their relatives, should be the responsibility of local authorities even if data for identification were obtained by international expert teams, as was the case during the investigation of the victims of the Southeast Asian tsunami disaster of 2005. Determination of the cause and manner of death by independent forensic experts can produce valuable information for purposes of local or international courts of law, and for national and international communities.

Clarification of the circumstances surrounding death is the element that probably draws the most public attention. Determination of these circumstances is not always possible due to, for example, postmortem changes. Moreover, in incidents of alleged political or ethnic violence, various versions concerning the course of events can exist, including a great deal of propaganda and incorrect conclusions (Rainio and Turunen, 2006). On the basis of forensic investigations, some of these versions can often be excluded, allowing investigators to at least conclude what had not happened (Rainio et al., 2001b; Rainio, 2001c). However, the role of the forensic scientist is not to judge the case, but to present evidence to be used in court (Rasmussen et al., 1990; Schäfer, 2000).

In forensic investigations of alleged political or ethnic violence, great objectivity and independency are required. Hence, for the benefit of the investigation, in some cases engaging the services of only independent experts, regardless of the professional level of the local experts, is advisable (Rainio, 2002). Furthermore, the independence of a forensic expert team requires a high level of proficiency and self-sufficiency in materials (Rainio et al., 2001b).

LEGAL FRAMEWORK

Request for Investigation

Depending on the situation, the organisation and legal framework in which the forensic expert teams have investigated victims of alleged political or ethnic violence have varied. Usually, forensic expert teams performing such investigations operate at governmental request, under the mandate of intergovernmental organisations, such as the United Nations (UN), European Union (EU), World Health Organization (WHO), or the United Nations Educational, Scientific and Cultural Organisation (UNESCO) (Snow et al., 1984; Rasmussen et al., 1990; United Nations 1995; Vanezis, 1999; Eriksson et al., 2000; Rainio et al., 2001a; Rainio, 2002), or at the request of non-governmental organisations, including the International Committee for the Red Cross, Physicians for Human Rights, Amnesty International or the Human Rights Watch (Snow et al., 1984; Thomsen et al., 1984; Kirschner and Hannibal, 1994; Brkic et al., 1997; Chandrasiri, 1997; Vanezis, 1999; Brkic et al., 2000; Schmitt, 2002; Simmons, 2002; Skinner et al., 2002). Legal representatives of the victims' families may also request an investigation (Vanezis, 1999).

Many countries have experienced forensic mass disaster investigations at a national or international level. The procedure used in mass disaster investigation can also be applied in a forensic expert operation after alleged political or ethnic violence (Thomsen et al., 1984; Stanković et al., 1994; Brkic et al., 2000; Lorin de la Grandmaison and Durigon, 2001). Previous experiences in mass disaster investigation can improve cooperation within the team in unusual working circumstances (Rainio, 2002).

Investigation of victims of an alleged mass violence, or victims from an alleged mass grave differs, however, from investigation of victims of a mass disaster in the cause and manner of death, and the condition and

number of victims. In addition, identification methods may diverge because of the differing availability of antemortem data. The mandate for
and the possibilities of the experts, and the expectations as to the results of investigation of a mass disaster or mass violence can also vary
markedly.

In a mass disaster, identification and cause-of-death investigations of
victims are generally conducted by local authorities, according to the
jurisdiction of the country in which the disaster occurs, although identification can be achieved only through close cooperation with the authorities of the victims' countries of residence (Interpol, 1992; Lunetta et
al., 2003).

Legal Issues

Several legal issues should be taken into account in the planning of
forensic expert team investigations in a foreign country (Rainio et al.,
2001a). If the team is established by the international community of
states, the mandate of the team and reasons for its creation normally involve several questions of public international law. These may include,
inter alia, the nature of investigative acts and issues relating to the com-
petence and powers of the initiating intergovernmental organisation, especially when the team is to function in a state which is not a member
of that particular organisation (Rasmussen et al., 1990; Vanezis, 1999;
Rainio et al., 2001a; Rainio, 2002).

Agreement must be reached in advance with local authorities that the
forensic expert team is formally permitted to operate in a certain area
(Rasmussen et al., 1990; Vanezis, 1999; Rainio et al., 2001a). The aims
set forth for the team in its mandate may include possible use of the results as part of factual evidence in later legal proceedings on a regional,
national, or international level. Then, if the particular tribunal already
exists, the team must take into consideration the requirements set forth
in the tribunal's rules of evidence in planning on-site activities and deciding on issues relating to the chain of custody (Rainio et al., 2001a;
Rainio, 2002). Usually, the team operates in the area of a sovereign
state. This means that the team has to take into account the legislation
of that state if the area is not under international supervision, or if the
team is not functioning on the basis of an obliging resolution of the UN
Security Council (Vanezis, 1999; Rainio et al., 2001a). The requirements
set forth in the legislation may also be partially or fully set aside in an

agreement concluded between the team or its home state and the government of the host state. The legislation of the host state may include strict rules, for instance, on the opening of graves, even at temporary burial sites, on treatment of human remains, and on reporting of findings (Vanezis, 1999; Rainio et al., 2001a; Rainio, 2002).

In forensic practice, principles concerning the concealment of personal information related to the individuals investigated, the official confirmation of victims' identity, and the division of duties between authorities, can vary significantly by country. Therefore, agreement should also be reached on these issues in advance.

Moreover, with a view to any ensuing legal actions, the status of team members should be elucidated. This includes each member's status in his or her capacity as a team member to perform the official functions of the team, as well as his or her civil and criminal responsibility in a private capacity as an individual performing legally valid acts in a foreign state (Rainio et al., 2001a; Rainio, 2002).

ORGANISATION

Advance Preparations

Crucial to the successful realisation of the operation and the avoidance of unrealistic expectations is that the mandate and the tasks of the forensic expert team are clearly defined before the operation commences. Furthermore, at this same stage, the detail in which the victims are to be examined should be determined.

The advance work in the operations carried out by the Finnish expert teams has included preparation of exhumation and autopsy equipment, briefing of personnel, and development of the investigative strategy and logistics (Rainio et al., 2001a).

In addition, advance preparations include safeguarding the health status of team members. According to recommendations of the Finnish National Public Health Institute regarding vaccination for the Balkan region, based on information from the WHO, the members of the Finnish UN-FET and EU-FET were vaccinated against hepatitis A and B, poliomyelitis, tetanus, diphtheria, tuberculosis, typhoid fever, rabies, meningococcal meningitis and epidemic encephalitis, if they had not already received these vaccinations (Rainio et al., 2001a). Forensic expert teams have usually been vaccinated against these diseases, except perhaps the latter two, and should also be protected against staphylococcal and streptococcal infections and enteritis (Skinner, 1987; Holck, 2000). In some FET operations, local authorities have required that the experts present a medical certificate.

Personal Security

Personal security of team members is a key condition, but it is not always ensured (Kirschner and Hannibal, 1994; Chandrasiri, 1997; Vanezis, 1999; Rainio et al., 2001a; Rainio et al., 2001b). Security at sites is also an important aspect of the chain of custody (Skinner 1987; Skinner and Lazenby, 1983; United Nations, 1995). Plans for security should include, *inter alia*, insurance, travel, housing and safe transportation during the operation. Moreover, it is essential to formulate a plan for evacuation of team members if the situation in the area rapidly deteriorates. Such plans should include provisions for transportation, protection and storage of equipment and samples taken and, in the case of evacuation, their safe preservation in the area of operation, if they cannot be withdrawn together with the team.

Concerning on-site security, paths in the field being investigated and all human remains and related items collected for examination are advised to be secured by explosive experts, who can also check all foreign objects during autopsies (Rainio et al., 2001a).

Exhumation and Autopsy Equipment

In all missions covered by the Finnish teams, the equipment necessary for exhumations was transported from Finland to ensure technical independence. This comprised the mine clearing officer's personal equipment, including special shoes, helmet and mine detector, shovels, axes, trowels, meter tape and measuring roll, isolation tape, writing and drawing materials and plates, plastic envelopes, body bags, carrying straps, bullet proof vests, first-aid kits with bandaging materials, salt solutions and antibacterial and analgesic drugs, documentation equipment and clothing for the team members. The latter included, for example, winter wool stockings. Forensic expert teams often work in difficult circumstances, both in the autopsy room and in the field.

Despite the intention, the Finnish teams never performed exhumations of single or mass graves in the territory of the former Yugoslavia, but examined human remains collected in the field, or previously exhumed bodies (Rainio et al., 2001a; Rainio et al., 2001c; Rainio et al., 2001d; Rainio, 2002). However, international forensic expert teams, also involving Finnish experts, have carried out exhumations of alleged single and mass graves in the former Yugoslavia, as shown in Figure 3-1.

Similar to the exhumation equipment, all equipment for autopsies was brought from Finland. This equipment included an accumulator and a compressor, an electric and a pneumatic circular saw, spare blades, autopsy tools and their sharpening equipment, probes, measuring sticks, magnifying glasses, tubes and bottles for the samples, cassettes for histological samples, necessary chemicals, forms to record postmortem findings, writing and drawing materials and mini-cassette recorders for dictating autopsy reports, clothing, masks, gloves and boots for the autopsy room, tools for the forensic odontologist's investigations and measuring equipment for the physical anthropologist's investigations (Rainio et al., 2001a). In addition, all necessary equipment for adequate DNA analysis sampling must be transported. Sampling may also be necessary in field conditions. Figure 3-2 shows a situation,

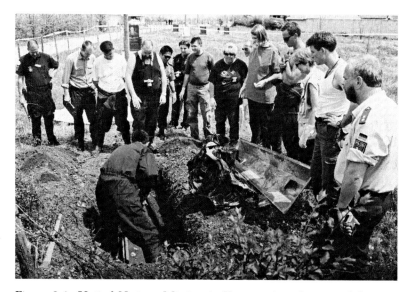

Figure 3-1. United Nations Mission in Kosovo. A multinational forensic team investigating a grave. (Photo: Ismo Kopra, Head of Exhumation Team, United Nations Mission in Kosovo).

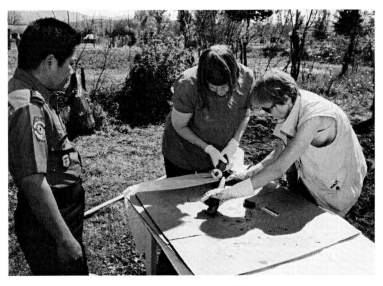

Figure 3-2. Sampling long bone tissue for DNA analysis in field conditions. (Photo: Ismo Kopra, Head of Exhumation Team, United Nations Mission in Kosovo).

in which the exhumations were performed in order to take DNA samples only. After that the bodies were reburied.

Personnel

The number of experts and their fields of specialisation, and the number of other personnel required, depends on the number and condition of the victims, on information surrounding the events, on tasks of the investigation, on the time period reserved for the operation and on many other factors (Morse et al., 1976; Boyd, 1979; Kirschner and Hannibal, 1994; Ludes et al., 1994; Chandrasiri, 1997; Vanezis, 1999; Rainio et al., 2001a). In medicolegal investigations of mass disasters and victims from mass graves, the forensic experts involved represent the following disciplines: forensic pathology, forensic anthropology, forensic genetics and forensic odontology. Moreover, forensic investigators, photographers, autopsy technicians, x-ray technicians, archaeologists, radiologists and forensic toxicologists, as well as site security, secretarial and logistic personnel are necessarily involved, and occasionally also entomologists and botanists (Morse et al., 1976; Boyd, 1979; Snow et al., 1984; Skinner, 1987; Griffiths and Oettle, 1993; Belyayev et al., 1994;

Kirschner and Hannibal, 1994; Ludes et al., 1994; Stanković et al., 1994; Boles et al., 1995; Blewitt, 1997; Brkic et al., 1997; Chandrasiri, 1997; Vanezis, 1999; Brkic et al., 2000; Holck, 2000; Rainio et al., 2001a; Rainio et al., 2001d). Since nearly all questions in the establishment and operation of a forensic expert team involve legal aspects, it would be beneficial for a team to have access to sufficient legal information and expertise.

PERFORMANCE

Exhumation Procedure

The course of action during exhumation is widely discussed in the literature (Morse et al., 1976; Bass and Birkby, 1978; Boyd, 1979; Skinner and Lazenby, 1983; Krogman and İşcan, 1986; Skinner, 1987; Knight, 1991; Griffiths and Oettle, 1993; Belyayev et al., 1994; Kirschner and Hannibal, 1994; United Nations, 1995). Detailed advance preparation is crucial for preservation of evidence during excavation of remains. The investigated area and the gravesite should be mapped, photographed and videotaped to demonstrate the location of the human remains in the area; scale and magnetic north should also be indicated (Morse et al., 1976; Bass and Birkby, 1978; Boyd, 1979; Krogman and İşcan, 1986; Skinner, 1987). At every stage, the exhumation procedure itself should be documented accurately, providing the scale and an identifying number for each of the remains or items (Skinner and Lazenby, 1983; Haglund et al., 1990; Knight, 1991; Kirschner and Hannibal, 1994). The position of the human remains at the site, as well as the orientation of the items and the relationship between different individuals and items must be apparent (Morse et al., 1976; Bass and Birkby, 1978; Skinner and Lazenby, 1983; Krogman and İşcan, 1986; Skinner, 1987; Chandrasiri, 1997; Vanezis, 1999). All findings made during the excavation should be recorded minutely *in situ* (Morse et al., 1976; Skinner, 1987; Haglund et al., 1990; Knight, 1991; Vanezis, 1999). Negative findings may also be informative (Knight, 1991). The main tasks in this process are the reconstruction of the events surrounding the burial, and the collection of all information that appears useful for determination of the cause and manner of death and for identification of the victims (Bass and Birkby, 1978; Skinner, 1987; Kirschner and Hannibal, 1994; Chandrasiri, 1997).

Transportation

Specific requirements for transportation include ensuring that human remains and other evidence are unharmed, and preventing any contamination or confusion (Dunne and McMeekin, 1977; Boyd, 1979; Skinner and Lazenby, 1983; Howard et al., 1988; Haglund et al., 1990; Chandrasiri, 1997). To this end, and to maintain the chain of custody, each sample should be packaged separately, in individual resistant body bags whenever possible (Dunne and McMeekin, 1977; McMeekin, 1980; Skinner and Lazenby, 1983; Chandrasiri, 1997; Brkic et al., 2000), and each package should be sealed and identified both inside and outside (Morse et al., 1976; Dunne and McMeekin, 1977; Boyd, 1979; McMeekin, 1980; Skinner and Lazenby, 1983; Krogman and İşcan, 1986; Howard et al., 1988; Chandrasiri, 1997). Thereafter, the packages, as well as the entire collection, should be photographed before transportation and re-photographed upon arrival at the place of investigation (Howard et al., 1988).

Autopsy

Autopsies should be carried out using standard methods of forensic pathology, taking care to preserve the chain of custody. The extent to which the victims are to be investigated should be agreed upon in advance. This will depend on the number of victims and the number of experts, as well as on the conditions of the investigation, including the facilities available.

During the medicolegal autopsy, all three cavities of the body should be opened and examined, even if injuries are not present in every region. All injuries and the vitality of the injuries, as well as all pathological changes caused by diseases should be recorded. In cases of gunshot wounds, bullet track directions inside the body should be determined. Furthermore, the autopsy should also include sampling specimens for histological and forensic toxicological investigations (Adelson, 1974; Knight, 1991; Interpol, 1992; United Nations, 1995; Brinkmann, 1999). Without a full autopsy examination, the results may to some extent remain speculative. By using standard methods agreed upon in advance for all cases under investigation, a systematic and comprehensive examination is ensured (for further reading on this topic see Chapter 5 of this volume).

Advance preparations concerning the tasks and roles of each expert and the working instructions should be scrupulously performed to avoid future inconsistencies. A detailed working scheme is especially important when the experts come from several countries, since standards of forensic investigation and reporting vary between countries. Marked differences in investigative standards can lead to insufficient examinations. Therefore, the use of a model protocol, such as the one suggested by the UN (United Nations, 1991; United Nations, 1995), is advisable. Clearly written, concrete and detailed working instructions should be accessible to all experts throughout the investigation.

Within the UN, a manual on the effective prevention and investigation of extralegal, arbitrary and summary executions was prepared (United Nations, 1991). Furthermore, in 1993, guidelines and procedures for the conduct of inquiries by the UN into allegations of massacres were developed (United Nations, 1995). These documents include a model autopsy protocol, a guide for postmortem detection of torture, and a model protocol for disinterment and analysis of skeletal remains. The model autopsy protocol is intended to have several applications. Firstly, it can be followed by experienced forensic pathologists to ensure systematic examinations and to facilitate meaningful positive or negative criticism by later observers. Secondly, general pathologists or other physicians may use the model protocol to supplement their customary autopsy procedures. Thirdly, this protocol has been proposed as the minimum criterion for actions or opinions of independent consultants or other representatives who may be requested to observe the autopsies. Historians, journalists and representatives of the public may also use it as a benchmark for evaluating an autopsy. Finally, it is intended for governments or individuals attempting to establish or upgrade their medicolegal systems (United Nations, 1991; United Nations, 1995). The model autopsy protocol includes sections on scene investigation, general conditions of the autopsy procedure, external and internal examination of the body, toxicological and histological investigations and documentation of the findings with photographs and x-rays.

Moreover, during various stages of the investigation, checking and re-checking that all data have been recorded according to the instructions assures standard results when experts with differing backgrounds are involved.

In searching for foreign objects, an x-ray examination should be conducted even in the case of skeletal remains, since the localisation of bullets or bullet fragments inside victims can be very challenging (Dutra, 1944; Fatteh and Mann, 1969; Evans and Knight, 1981; DiMaio, 1985; Dodd and Budzik, 1990; Messmer, 1998; Kahana and Hiss, 1999; Jacobs et al., 2000; Rainio et al., 2001e). Radiological methods should therefore be applied to determine and document the existence, number, localisation and identification of foreign material inside victims (Fatteh and Mann, 1969; Adelson, 1974; Evans and Knight, 1981; Schmidt and Kallieris, 1982; DiMaio, 1985; Dodd and Budzik, 1990; Hollerman et al., 1990; Messmer, 1998). Estimation of retained bullets and, consequently, determination of exact entrance and exit wounds can be difficult without radiology in cases of multiple gunshot wounds. The application of fluoroscopy in screening foreign objects and gross bone injuries should be considered in mass disasters and investigations of atrocities with high numbers of casualties (Fitzpatrick, 1984; Chandrasiri, 1997; Jacobs et al., 2001).

The results of forensic toxicological analysis can clarify the background, or sometimes even the course of events leading to death, even in cases with a long postmortem interval (Grellner and Glenewinkel, 1997).

DNA analysis has been increasingly applied in international and national forensic investigations (Rainio et al., 2001d; Budowle et al., 2005). Since the primary motivation for DNA analysis is the identification of individuals, and since the sampling is often performed during autopsy by forensic personnel not specialised in this area, basic knowledge of DNA identification and its caveats is important. The general issues and guidelines for (1) reference and case sample collection, preservation, shipping and storage, (2) chain of custody and tracking of data, (3) DNA typing laboratory facilities, including quality assurance and quality control, (4) DNA analysis, including DNA extraction, DNA typing and interpretation of results, automation and software issues, and (5) handling of information concerning families and relatives involved and the associated privacy issues have to be clear to all investigators involved, and established before the DNA identification process is started. In addition, careful selection of reference population databases and matching criteria by DNA specialists will optimise the use of DNA for identification purposes.

While in the field, unnecessary biological material taken during an autopsy can be (re)buried along with the body from which it was removed. What is clear is that this type of material should be destroyed or disposed of according to local instructions, which can vary depending on the country where the work is being conducted. On the other hand, when autopsy samples need to be examined later on, as the Finnish Team has done during prior missions, the material is treated in Finland as hazardous waste; however, histological samples imbedded in paraffin blocks were filed and kept as part of all the documentation pertaining to the investigation.

During the final period of the Račak investigation, when the Finnish forensic pathologists were writing their executive reports, experimental shooting of living animals was deemed necessary (Rainio et al., 2001c; Rainio et al., 2003). This action was required to confirm the conclusions drawn in Kosovo, and it proved useful because gunshot injuries inflicted by military weapons are rare in Finland. This experiment led to more accurate judgements concerning wounds seen in Kosovo.

Documentation

An important requirement for documenting the investigation is clear and unambiguous reports produced by experts, including an explanation of the chain of custody during the investigation. A consecutive summary, integrating the results of pathologists, anthropologists, geneticists, odontologists and other experts can facilitate comprehension of the report.

Radiological methods, together with photographs and video recording produce illustrative documentation (Fatteh and Mann, 1969; Adelson, 1974; Tedeshi, 1984; Hooft et al., 1989; Ludes et al., 1994; United Nations, 1995; Jacobs et al., 2000; Rainio et al., 2001a; Rainio, 2002). This documentation complements the autopsy reports, as well as the reports of forensic anthropologists, forensic archaeologists, forensic odontologists, forensic geneticists, and other experts. Radiological data, photographs, and video films can also be used in court, and in situations where people not present during the investigation need to be briefed (see Chapters 5 and 6 of this volume).

In medicolegal investigation of mass disasters or mass graves, photographs and videotapes are useful for both identification and documentation. For identification, antemortem photographs can also be of value (Cornwell, 1956; Sosedko and Lavrentyuk, 1995; Brkic et al., 2000). Photographic and video documentation of medicolegal investigations has several requirements. At each site to be examined, the entire investigatory area should first be photographed and videofilmed, including aerial views whenever possible (Morse et al., 1976; Boyd, 1979; Skinner and Lazenby, 1983; Krogman and İşcan, 1986; Haglund et al., 1990; United Nations, 1995). The recovery of victims should then be carefully photographed and video filmed. Autopsy photographs should include front and side views of the face, general views of all sides of the body, clothed and unclothed, and close-up views of the injuries and other findings, with a scale to provide a size reference (Fisher, 1973; Dunne and McMeekin, 1977; Boyd, 1979; Tedeschi, 1984; Knight, 1991; Sosedko and Lavrentyuk, 1995; United Nations, 1995; Brinkmann, 1999). In every photograph, the autopsy number must be visible, and in close-up pictures, also a scale indicating the particular wound or other finding (Hooft et al., 1989; United Nations, 1995; Chandrasiri, 1997).

Reporting and Filing

Naturally, the reporting depends on the preferences of the instigator of the forensic investigation, and on the ultimate purpose of the operation. The official reporting of results should be decided in advance. The commissioner of the investigation can distribute the reports circumspectly, or make the results public. The investigation may receive national or international attention, but the privacy of the victims and their relatives must not be forgotten. In addition, use of and access to the materials, for example, for scientific purposes should be clarified. Furthermore, the chain of custody should be considered when deciding where to permanently store the autopsy protocols, photographs, samples and other documents after the team's work has concluded. The Finnish teams filed master copies of all documents at the Institute of Forensic Medicine, University of Helsinki, including any histological samples imbedded in paraffin blocks.

SUMMARY

International missions for investigation of alleged human rights violations often involve forensic experts. Several legal and practical aspects should be taken into consideration when a forensic expert team is prepared for such a mission. These aspects include the mandate of the team to operate in a sovereign state, material independency of the team, personal security of team members, clear instructions for exhumation and autopsy procedures, documentation of the investigation and findings and reporting of results. To ensure successful realisation of the mission, these matters should be agreed upon in advance.

REFERENCES

Adelson, L. (1974). *The pathology of homicide.* Springfield: Charles C Thomas.

Bass, W.M., and Birkby, W.H. (1978). Exhumation: The method could make the difference. *FBI Law Enforcement Bull:* 6–11.

Belyayev, L.V., Granenov, V.M., Radevich, S.S., Tretetsky, A.V., Shalamaev, S.V., and Yablokov, A.Y. (1994). О работе комиссии российско-польских экспертов по эксгумации трупов польских военнопленных. (Activities of commission of Russian and Polish experts on exhumation of corpses of Polish prisoners of war. In Russian) *Sudebnomeditsinskaja expertiza, 37*: 37–40.

Blewitt, G.T. (1997). The role of forensic investigations in genocide prosecutions before an international criminal tribunal. *Med Sci Law, 37*: 284–288.

Boles, T.C., Snow, C.C., and Stover, E. (1995). Forensic DNA testing on skeletal remains from mass graves: Pilot project in Guatemala. *J Forensic Sci, 40*: 349–355.

Boyd, R.M. (1979). Buried body cases. *FBI Law Enforcement Bull:* 1–7.

Brinkmann, B. (1999). Harmonisation of medico-legal autopsy rules. *Int J Legal Med, 113*: 1–14.

Brkic, H., Strinović, D., Kubat, M., and Petrovecki, V. (2000). Odontological identification of human remains from mass graves in Croatia. *Int J Legal Med, 114*: 19–22.

Brkic, H., Strinović, D., Vlaus, M., Skavić, J., Zevević, D., and Milicevic, M. (1997). Dental identification of war victims from Petrinja in Croatia. *Int J Legal Med, 110*: 47–51.

Budowle, B., Bieber, F.R., and Eisenberg, A.J. (2005). Forensic aspects of mass disaster: Strategic considerations for DNA-based human identification. *Legal Med, 7*: 230–243.

Chandrasiri, N. (1997). Experiences of a forensic pathologist in the examination of a mass grave in Former Yugoslavia. *Ceylon Med J, 42*: 98–102.

Cordner, S., and McKelvie, H. (1998). Forensic medicine: international criminal tribunals and an International Criminal Court. *Lancet, 351*: 1956–1957.

Cordner, S., and Ranson, D.L. (1997). Grim new role for forensic pathologist. *Lancet, 350* (suppl III): 6.

Cornwell, W.S. (1956). Radiography and photography in problems of identification: A review. *Med Radiography Photography, 32*: 1, 34–35.

Dillner, L. (1994). Human rights group condemns UN in Rwanda. *BMJ, 309:* 895.

DiMaio, V.J.M. (1985). *Gunshot wounds.* New York, Elsevier.

Dodd, G.D. III, and Budzik, R.F., Jr. (1990). Identification of retained firearm projectiles on plain radiographs. *Am J Roentgen, 154*: 471–475.

Dunne, M.J., and McMeekin, R.R. (1977). Medical investigation of fatalities from aircraft-accident burns. *Aviat Space Environ Med:* 964–968.

Dutra, F.R. (1944). Identification of person and determination of cause of death from skeletal remains. *Arch Pathol, 38*:339–349.

Eriksson, A., Hougen, H.P., Knudsen, P.T., Leth, P., Lynnerup, N., and Sprogøe-Jakobsen, S. (2000). Dansk-Svenskt Rättsmedicinskt Arbete i Kosovo 1999, II. Rättsmedicinska Fynd och Erfarenheter (Danish-Swedish forensic pathology teams in Kosovo 1999, II. Examination and identification of war crime victims. (In Swedish). *Nordisk Rettsmedisin, 3*: 4–79.

Evans, K.T., and Knight, B. (1981). *Forensic radiology.* Oxford: Blackwell.

Fatteh, A.V., and Mann, G.T. (1969). The role of radiology in forensic pathology. *Med Sci Law, 9*:27–30.

Ferllini, R. (2003). The development of human rights investigations since 1945. *Sci Justice, 43*:21.

Fisher, R.S. (1973). Aircraft crash investigation. In *Medicolegal Investigation of Death.* Spitz, W.U. and Fisher, R.S. (Eds.). Springfield, Charles C Thomas, pp. 347–359.

Fitzpatrick, J.J. (1984). Role of radiology in human rights abuse. *Am J Forensic Med Path, 5*:321–325.

Geiger, H.J. (1996). Balkan war crimes indictment. *Lancet, 347*:672.

Grellner, W., and Glenewinkel, F. (1997). Exhumations: Synopsis of morphological and toxicological findings in relation to the postmortem interval. Survey on a 20-Year Period and Review of the Literature. *Forensic Sci Int, 90*:139–159.

Griffiths, C.J.G., and Oettle, T.H.G. (1993). Forensic odontology in war graves exhumation in the Ukraine. *J Forensic Odonto-Stomat, 11*:63–69.

Gunby, P. (1994). Medical team seeks to identify human remains from mass graves of war in Former Yugoslavia. *JAMA, 272*: 1804–1806.

Haglund, W.D. (2002). Recent mass graves, an introduction. In *Advances in forensic taphonomy: Method, theory, and archaeological perspectives,* Haglund, W.D., and Sorg, M.H. (Eds.). Boca Raton: CRC Press, pp. 243–261.

Haglund, W.D., Reichert, D.G., and Reay, D.T. (1990). Recovery of decomposed and skeletal human remains in the "Green River Murder" investigation. *Am J Forensic Med Path, 11*:35–43.

Hill, I.R., Howell, R.D., and Jarmulowicz, M. (1988). Identification in the Manchester air disaster. *Brit Dent J*:445–446.

Holck, P. (2000). Erfaringer fra Kosovo (Experiences from Kosovo. In Danish). *Nordisk rettsmedisin, 3*:66–68.

Hollerman, J.J., Fackler, M.L., Coldwell, D.M., and Ben-Menachem, Y. (1990). Gunshot wounds: 2. Radiology. *Am J Roentgenol, 155*:691–702.

Hooft, P.J., Noji, E.K., and van de Voorde, H.P. (1989). Fatality management in mass casualty incidents. *Forensic Sci Int, 40*:3–14.

Howard, J.D., Reay, D.T., Haglund, W.D., and Fligner, C.L. (1988). Processing of skeletal remains. A medical examiner's perspective. *Am J Forensic Med Path, 9*:258–264.

Interpol (1992). *Manual on disaster victim identification.* Paris: International Criminal Police Organization.

Jacobs, W., Campobasso, C., and Dewinne, J. (2000). Organisational aspects of disaster victim identification (DVI) work: Lessons from the exhumation, examination and human identification of war graves in the Former Yugoslavia (Kosovo). *Ann Med Milit Belg, 14*:193–197.

Jacobs, W., Hermans, W., Campobasso, C., and Dewinne, J. (2001). Ballistic trauma analysis of 212 victims recovered from 6 mass graves in the former Yugoslavia. *Ann Med Milit Belg, 15*:11–14.

Kahana, T., Freund, M., and Hiss, J. (1997). Suicidal terrorist bombings in Israel - Identification of human remains. *J Forensic Sci, 42*:260–264.

Kahana, T., and Hiss, J. (1999). Forensic radiology. *Brit J Radiology, 72*:129–133.

Kirschner, R.H., and Hannibal, K.E. (1994). The application of the forensic sciences to human rights investigations. *Med Law, 13*:451–460.

Knight, B. (1991). *Forensic pathology.* London: Edward Arnold.

Krogman, W.M., and Iscan, M.Y. (1986). *The human skeleton in forensic medicine.* Springfield: Chales C Thomas.

Kuzman, M., Tomic, B., Stevanovic, R., Ljubicic, M., Katalinic, D., and Rodin, U. (1993). Fatalities in the war in Croatia, 1991 and 1992: Underlying and external causes of death. *JAMA, 270*:626–628.

Lorin de la Grandmaison, G., and Durigon, M. (2001). Do medico-legal truths have more power than war lies? About the conflicts in the Former Yugoslavia and Kosovo. *Med Sci Law, 41*:301–304.

Ludes, B., Tracqui, A., Pfitzinger, H., Kintz, P., Levy, F., Disteldorf, M., Hutt, J.M., Kaess, B., Haag, R., Memheld, B., Kaempf, C., Friederich, F., Evenot, E., and Mangin, P. (1994). Medico-legal investigation of the airbus A320 crash upon Mount Ste-Odile, France. *J Forensic Sci, 39*:1147–1152.

Lunetta, P., Ranta, H., Cattaneo, C., Piccinini, A., Niskanen, R., Sajantila, A., and Penttilä, A. (2003). International collaboration in mass disasters involving foreign nationals within the EU. Medico-legal investigation of Finnish victims of the Milan Linate Airport SAS SK 686 aircraft accident on 8 October 2001. *Int J Legal Med, 117*:204–210.

Macilwain, C. (1995). Forensic team digs up Haiti's deadly past. *Nature, 377:* 278.

Marcikić, M., Kraus, Z., Dmitrović, B., Zibar, L., Matković, S., and Marušić, A. (1993). View of a war from a pathology department: Croatian experience. *Med and War, 9*: 33–39.

McMeekin, R.R. (1980). An organizational concept for pathologic identification in mass disasters. *Aviat Space Environ Med*: 999–1003.

Messmer, J.M. (1998). Radiology of gunshot wounds. In *Forensic Radiology*, Brogdon, B.G. (Ed.). Boca Raton: CRC Press, pp. 209–223.

Morse, D., Crusoe, D., and Smith, H.G. (1976). Forensic archaeology. *J Forensic Sci, 21*:323–332.

Petersen, H.D., and Vedel, O.M. (1994). Assessment of evidence of human rights violations in Kashmir. *Forensic Sci Int, 68*:103–115.

Primorac, D., Andelinović, S., Definis-Gojanović, M., Drmic, I., Rezic, B., Baden, M.M., Kennedy, M.A., Schanfield, M.S., Skakel, S.B., and Lee, H.C. (1996). Identification of war victims from mass graves in Croatia, Bosnia, and Herzegovina by the use of standard forensic methods and DNA typing. *J Forensic Sci, 41*: 891–894.

Rainio, J. (2002). *Independent forensic examination of victims of armed conflict: investigations of Finnish forensic expert teams in the Balkan area.* Academic Dissertation. Helsinki, Yliopistopaino.

Rainio, J., Lalu, K., Ranta, H., Takamaa, K., and Penttilä, A. (2001a). Practical and legal aspects of forensic autopsy expert team operations. *Legal Med, 4*:220–232.

Rainio, J., Karkola, K., Lalu, K., Ranta, H., Takamaa, K., and Penttilä A. (2001b). Forensic investigations in Kosovo: Experiences of the European Union forensic expert team. *J Clin Forensic Med, 8*:218–221.

Rainio, J., Lalu, K., and Penttilä, A. (2001c). Independent forensic autopsies in an armed conflict - investigation of the victims from Racak, Kosovo. *Forensic Sci Int, 116*(2,3):171–185.

Rainio, J., Hedman, M., Karkola, K., Lalu, K., Peltola, P., Ranta, H., Sajantila, A., Söderholm, N., and Penttilä, A. (2001d). Forensic osteological investigations in Kosovo. *Forensic Sci Int, 121*:169–177.

Rainio, J., Lalu, K., Ranta, H., and Penttilä, A. (2001e). Radiology in forensic expert team operations. *Legal Med, 3*:34–43.

Rainio, J., Lalu, K., Ranta, H., and Penttilä, A. (2003). Morphology of experimental assault rifle skin wounds. *Int J Legal Med, 117*:19–26.

Rainio, J., and Turunen, M. (2006). The examination and reporting on war crimes – An example from Finnish history. *Int J Legal Med, 120*:89–94.

Ranta, H., and Penttilä, A. (1999). Finnish forensic expert team in Bosnia and Herzegovina. In *The Finnish Yearbook of International Law*, Koskenniemi, M. (Ed.). The Hague: Kluwer Law International and Ius Gentium Association, pp. 420–431.

Rasmussen, O.V., Helweg-Larsen, K., Kelstrup, J., Carlé, P., and Rehof, L.A. (1990). The medical component in fact-finding missions. *Dan Med Bull, 37*:371–374.

Schäfer, A.Th. (2000). Rectsmedizinische Erfahrungen im Kosovo. (Forensic medicine experiences in Kosovo. In German) *Arch Kriminol, 205*:110–116.

Schmidt, G., and Kallieris, D. (1982). Use of radiographs in the forensic autopsy. *Forensic Sci Int, 19*:263–270.

Schmitt, S. (2002). Mass graves and the collection of forensic evidence: Genocide, war crimes, and crimes against humanity. In *Advances in forensic taphonomy: Method, theory, and archaeological perspectives*, Haglund, W.D., and Sorg, M.H. (Eds.). Boca Raton: CRC Press, pp. 277–292.

Simmons, T. (2002). Taphonomy of a karstic cave execution site at Hrgar, Bosnia-Herzegovina. In *Advances in forensic taphonomy: Method, theory, and archaeological perspectives*, Haglund, W.D., and Sorg, M.H. (Eds.). Boca Raton: CRC Press, pp. 263–276.

Skinner, M. (1987). Planning the archaeological recovery of evidence from recent mass graves. *Forensic Sci Int, 34*:267–287.

Skinner, M., and Lazenby, R.A. (1983). *Found! human remains. A field manual for the recovery of the recent human skeleton*. Burnaby, BC: Archaeology Press, Simon Fraser University.

Skinner, M., York, H.P., and Connor, M.A. (2002). Postburial disturbance of graves in Bosnia-Herzegovina. In *Advances in forensic taphonomy: Method, theory, and archaeological perspectives*, Haglund, W.D., and Sorg, M.H. (Eds.). Boca Raton: CRC Press, pp. 293–308.

Skolnick, A.A. (1995). Forensic scientists helping Haiti heal. *JAMA, 274*:1181–1182.

Snow, C.C., Tedeschi, L.G., Levine, L., Orrego, C., Lukash, L., and Stover, E. (1984). The investigation of the human remains of the "disappeared" in Argentina. *Am J Forensic Med Path, 5*:297–299.

Sosedko, Y.I., and Lavrentyuk, G.P. (1995). Организация работы военных судебно-медицинских экспертов по опознанию погибших в зоне вооруженного конфликта. (Organisation of work of military legal physicians in identification of perished in the zone of armed conflict. In Russian). *Vojenno-meditsinskij žurnal, 6:* 24–26.

Sprogøe-Jakobsen, S., Eriksson, A., Hougen, H.P., Knudsen, P.J.T., Leth, P., and Lynnerup, N. (2001). Mobile autopsy teams in the investigation of war crimes in Kosovo 1999. *J Forensic Sci, 46:*1392–1396.

Stanković, Z. (1992). Sudsko-medicinska ekspertiza dvadeset četvoro ubijenih građana iz Gospiča okoline grada (Forensic-medical expertise of twenty-four murdered citizens from Gospič and its surroundings). *Vojnosanitetski pregled, 49:*143–170.

Stover, E. (1985). Scientists aid search for Argentina's 'desaparecidos'. *Science, 230:*56–57.

Strinović, D., Kostovic, I., Heningsberg, N., Judas, M., and Clark, D. (1994). Identification of war victims in Croatia. *Med Sci Law, 34:* 207–212.

Tedeschi, L.G. (1984). Methodology in the forensic sciences. Documentation of human rights abuses. *Am J Forensic Med Path, 5:* 301–303.

Thomsen, J.L., Gruschow, J., and Stover, E. (1989). Medicolegal investigation of political killings in El Salvador. *Lancet, 1:* 1377–1379.

Thomsen, J.L., Helweg-Larsen, K., and Rasmussen, O.V. (1984). Amnesty International and the forensic sciences. *Am J Forensic Med Path, 5:* 305–311.

United Nations (1957). *Standard minimum rules for the treatment of prisoners.* New York: United Nations, Economic and Social Council, Resolution 663 C (XXIV) of 31 July, 1957.

United Nations (1984a). *Safeguards guaranteeing protection of the rights of those facing the death penalty.* New York: United Nations, Economic and Social Council, Resolution 1984/50 of 25 May, 1984.

United Nations (1984b). *Convention against torture and other cruel, inhuman or degrading treatment or punishment, 10 December, 1984.* New York: United Nations, Treaty Series, Vol. 1465, p. 85.

United Nations (1989). *Effective prevention and investigation of extralegal, arbitrary and summary executions.* New York: United Nations, Economic and Social Council, Resolution 1989/65 of 24 May, 1989.

United Nations (1991). *Manual on the effective prevention and investigation of extra-legal, arbitrary and summary executions.* New York: United Nations, Centre for Social Development and Humanitarian Affairs, 1–72.

United Nations (1995). *Guidelines for the Conduct of United Nations inquiries into allegations of massacres.* New York: United Nations, Office of Legal Affairs, pp. 1–108.

van den Bos, A. (1980). Mass identification: A multidisciplinary operation. *Am J Forensic Med Path, 1:* 265–270.

Vanezis, P. (1997). Forensic pathology in a troubled world. *Med Sci Law, 37:* 277–283.

Vanezis, P. (1999). Investigation of clandestine graves resulting from human rights abuses. *J Clin Forensic Med, 6:* 238–242.

Woodhouse, T. (1999). Preventive medicine: Can conflicts be prevented? The evidence suggests that conflict prevention can work. *BMJ, 319:* 396–397.

Zečević, D., Škavić, J., Strinović, D., Gusić, S., Kubat, M., Čadež, J., and Marušić, A. (1993). Medical center for human rights. *Croatian Med J, 34:* 84–89.

Chapter 4

CRIME-SCENE MANAGEMENT AND FORENSIC ANTHROPOLOGY: OBSERVATIONS AND RECOMMENDATIONS FROM THE UNITED KINGDOM AND INTERNATIONAL CASES

CORINNE DUHIG AND RON TURNBULL

INTRODUCTION

The role of the Crime Scene Manager (CSM) includes technical aspects of crime scene investigation and evidence recovery, in addition to crucial leadership aspects such as assumption of responsibility, organisation and motivation of staff, proficient communication skills and responsibility for health and safety concerns (see for example, Pepper 2005, Chapter 10). Within these aspects, the specific use of one particular expert, the forensic anthropologist, will be primarily dealt with within this chapter.

Although the focus of this volume is on international cases, examples are included from our casework in the UK because it is possible to extrapolate from these to the conditions of the international mission. We refer to the Crime Scene Manager as "he" and the forensic anthropologist as "she" throughout: this is merely for convenience, reflecting our own areas of expertise, and is not intended to convey any gender-based division of roles. Additionally, the first and second author in this chapter will be referred as CD and RT respectively.

The expertise of a forensic anthropologist embraces what many refer to as "archaeology" and "anthropology" functions (see also below). For the first function, the determination of the non-forensic interest of bones is effected, through the planning and participation in searches, the excavation of single graves or recovery of surface remains, and the recording and clearance of mass graves in international operations. For the second, she can produce anthropological profiles of unidentified remains, assist the pathologist with the reconstruction of bodies and interpretation of antemortem and perimortem pathologies of the skeleton and trauma assessment; deal with cremated remains and – increasingly one of the most important functions – interpret the taphonomic history of bodies and their deposition sites (see Chapters 5 and 6 of this volume for further information on these topics).

There is sometimes, however, a lack of awareness in police circles of the anthropologist's potential contribution, even extending to complete ignorance that such a specialised job even exists. Anthropology overlaps to a lesser or greater extent with several other specialisms, which may cause difficulty and confusion for an inexperienced Senior Investigating Officer (SIO) or Crime Scene Manager (CSM) who has to plan the staffing of the investigation, in addition to co-ordinating all participants effectively at the scene. As the introduction of each additional specialist to a scene adds another opportunity for possible contamination, and the investigation cannot bear unlimited staffing costs, it might be unclear as to whether a forensic anthropologist should be called at all when other staff can be utilised. There could also be problems of management when a multiplicity of specialists are attending a scene, both in terms of demarcation and simple logistics, and the different backgrounds of all the internal and external staff may produce communication difficulties. This can be particularly acute when individuals are deployed on international missions, when working and living conditions are likely to be less than optimal and the usual stress of an investigation is increased manyfold by such factors as language difficulties, isolation, extreme fatigue, complicated logistics, and even physical danger. These three points – ignorance, overstaffing/role overlap and human-resources management challenges – will be elaborated below.

So far as is known, a forensic investigation has not collapsed as a result of the inappropriate use of forensic anthropology. Nevertheless, in our working lives we have observed numerous situations in which an improved understanding by the CSM of the background, strengths and weaknesses of the anthropological discipline would have optimised the results of a criminal investigation and the identification of the deceased.

We therefore make recommendations as to how the CSM should utilise anthropological expertise in the search and recovery of human remains, and their associated artefacts, and the interpretation of their depositional context. Furthermore, we see the interrelationship of the anthropologist and all other personnel at the scene as in need of informed and sensitive management by the CSM.

EDUCATION AND TRAINING OF FORENSIC ANTHROPOLOGISTS IN THE UK

Firstly, it is necessary to outline the structure of forensic-anthropological education and training in the UK at present, in order that the reader will understand the background of such specialists and, sometimes, the contrast with their colleagues from other countries. We use the classification as understood in the United States as our baseline, since this has been the source of most of our forensic training and protocols until recently. "Anthropology" within this terminology contains four disciplines:

- archaeology
- physical anthropology (now, changed to biological anthropology)
- social anthropology (cultural anthropology as it is known in many parts of the world)
- linguistics

In the UK, these subjects have tended to be divided between separate departments, often within separate faculties, with the first two in science and the second two in humanities. Increasingly, students may now combine archaeology and physical anthropology in their studies,[1] but this has not always been the case. The skills required for forensic anthropology emanate primarily from these two subjects, but if the practitioner has also studied social/cultural anthropology, she/he may be able to aid in interpretation of perpetrator behaviour, especially of a ritual nature, which might have ethnographic parallels: for example, CD has been asked to interpret the meaning of possible "witchcraft/black magic" hate-mailings in England. Additionally, burials as the result of

---

1. The first three have always been combined at Cambridge University, where CD chose to take her degree in the 1980s for this reason.

genocide may often include treatment meted to bodies that is intended to violate the victims' religion or culture. By contrast, some practitioners have come to forensic anthropology from a background of anatomy or medicine, and others have begun with a degree in forensic science and learned their anthropological skills through attaining a higher degree. Brickley and Ferllini (Brickley and Ferllini, 2007) discuss the training of forensic anthropologists in Europe, illustrating that UK practitioners have a limited number of institutions at their disposal in which anthropological or related education may be enhanced by forensic training, or where forensic science students may seek further courses in anthropology.

As mentioned above, there are two main facets to the anthropologist's work; fieldwork and mortuary functions. A few practitioners remain in one of these areas for their entire professional lives, particularly those who have already built up a very solid portfolio of work, and such individuals will be called only for that function. We believe, however, that because of the mutual feedback of these disciplines, and particularly because of the role of taphonomic interpretation, it is essential that both are conducted by one person or team, or that there exists an extremely close and regular communication between those in the two disciplines working on the same case.

Case Study: An Early Example

Many years ago, a train entered Edinburgh station in Scotland with a torso jammed between the couplings. As a young police officer with the local authorities and with no forensic training, RT was placed in a team which included volunteer members of the public. Attempts were made to locate the associated body parts, with the participants being equipped with simple bags, string and cardboard labels. Parts of the extremities were located beside the track, and were sent with the torso to the mortuary. Concurrently, another police force had located body parts beside the track nearer to the train's source,[2] and using similar methods, forwarded those body parts to the same mortuary. It took the forensic pathologist and his team a considerable time to establish that these were the commingled remains of two young men, and to confirm that many

---

2. For those who know Scotland, the first location was to the north of the Firth of Forth and the second to the south, near to the bridge.

body parts were still missing. However, the case was subsequently taken over by Special Branch (it was rumoured that the men were in Special Forces training), so it is not known whether further search was carried out to recover any more of the body parts. However, the commingling suggests that they fell from the train or got on to the track at the same point, and taphonomic factors (scavenger disturbance and continued train activity on the track were suggested) dispersed the remains over several miles. This would have been an ideal case for a forensic anthropologist, including field search and requiring specialised knowledge of anatomy and taphonomy. Unfortunately, in those days there were no forensic anthropologists at all practicing in the British Isles!

PROBLEM ONE: IGNORANCE

Even in the twenty-first century, usually the initial, and often only, contact a British police officer has with an anthropologist is when a member of the public walks into the police station with some bones in a sack or box, discovered whilst building an extension to their house or while digging in their garden or allotment. This is then brought to the attention of a CID officer (Criminal Investigation Department), whose responsibility it is to obtain the services of an individual who can inform him or her as to whether they are of forensic interest. Similarly, a body or body part may be discovered in abnormal circumstances, such as by surface exposure, shallow graves, in disused or burnt-out houses or washed up or dredged from a watercourse, and whilst these are obviously forensically significant, there is often some uncertainty as to who should advise on recovery and analysis and, particularly, on the interpretation of the depositional circumstances.

Only a few years ago most British police officers would undoubtedly have contacted a local pathologist first. Anthropologists in their forensic role were little known, not being mentioned in police training courses or manuals, and the pathologist was regarded as the expert as far as skeletons were concerned, being obviously the expert in the human body generally. With some exceptions however, pathologists, even forensic pathologists who dealt almost entirely with criminal cases and therefore bodies in various stages of decomposition, had received only rudimentary tuition pertaining to human skeletal anatomy, and few elaborated upon it much in later years. The average pathologist presented with human bones would not refer the police to an anthropologist but would offer a "guesstimate" as to the date and origin of the bones, perhaps because he or she had no contact with any anthropologists, because they felt they should take the responsibility for which they were retained or because of professional protectionism – some have been accused of arrogance but it is more likely to have been a combination of a genuine desire to help and the belief that they could provide the answers.

The situation can be complicated by the fact that the Coroner[3] is usually involved and might make his or her own assessment of who should be utilised in the investigation. In the absence of a pathologist, other persons might be called in instead; in very approximate order of usefulness, we know of cases in which the police or Coroner have involved a police surgeon as it is called in the UK, although now some prefer to be referred to as forensic medical examiners; a local archaeology unit, a hospital (non-forensic) pathologist, a local museum curator, a doctor, and a veterinarian.

At the scene, unlikely as it may seem, many CSMs in the UK have never worked on a clandestine burial investigation – in fact, one said of CD "I hope she knows more about homicide than I do." The forensic anthropologist is frequently the only person in an investigation other than the pathologist who works exclusively on death investigations. This is not so in the Metropolitan Police (Met), where RT was one of twelve detectives appointed solely as Homicide Advisors; other police services are now introducing the concept of Major Investigations Teams based upon the Met model.

By contrast, situations in which genocides and war crimes have been committed may result in the discovery of mass or single graves, and also surface scatter. The CSMs involved in such situations, whatever their background, will usually be affiliated with organisations such as the International Criminal Tribunal for the former Yugoslavia (ICTY), the International Criminal Tribunal for Rwanda (ICTR), the International Commision of Missing Persons (ICMP) and so on, and will be employed full-time or seconded for lengthy periods on mass grave investigations. They are likely be very familiar with the role of the

---

3. In England and Wales the Coroner (and the Procurator Fiscal in Scotland) has a unique role in death investigations, having jurisdiction over the body and its disposal which overrules any other persons' right, including those of the police investigators.

anthropologist, and if they are not they will, usually, become so rapidly in the intensive field conditions. Problems of management still remain however, as we discuss below.

Non-Forensic Remains

The "bread and butter" of most forensic anthropologists are cases in which skeletonised or semi-skeletonised remains are found unexpectedly and are in need of evaluation in order to determine whether or not they are of forensic interest.

The soil tends to be full of small bones of wild and domestic animals, birds, even lower vertebrates. Larger domestic food animals, and, in many countries, wild animals may also be found buried or as surface exposures. Osteological comparative anatomy is one of the key skills of the anthropologist, and this knowledge allows her to rapidly exclude any non-human bones at the scene. For example, whilst on a placement in the Balkans, CD advised RT that the few small bones found in a grave were those of a rabbit rather than the remains of a suspicious burial of an infant (which would have contradicted previous evidence and complicated the enquiry); other cases have included a cow skeleton in a "grave" beside a drainage ditch, probably illicitly buried during the foot-and-mouth crisis in England in 2001; dogs and cats in what appeared to be babies' graves, identified on the first sight of a bone beneath the wrappings rather than requiring full exhumation, and swan bones – large bones and fairly unfamiliar to most people – washed up from a watercourse. Unless there is some particular requirement for her to attend the scene immediately, CD now asks for digital photographs to be sent to her, and this usually enables her to identify animal bones without needing to attend – this is a method which the police find very convenient, saving time, money and deployment of a full major-incident team.

Of course, there is no special expertise required in order to identify the remains of the major food animals (for the UK this normally means pig, sheep/goat, cow, chicken and rabbit as food and dog, cat, small rodent and horse as domestic), at least when there is soft tissue preservation or the skeleton is well-preserved. Most people, though not all, are able to recognise the skulls of animals, at least as non-human, but it does require the attending officers to consider the possibility and to make appropriate enquiries before a full forensic team is called out.

Case Study: The Stolen Sheep

In the south of London, in the jurisdiction of the Metropolitan Police, a family had a barbeque in the garden of their new home and left food remains on the barbeque when they went inside in the evening. One of their guests returned to the garden later and saw body parts scattered across the lawn and protruding from what he described as a shallow grave. The local authorities were contacted, and a uniformed police officer arrived at the alleged scene; using her torch to view the scene from the opposite end of the garden she concluded that it was a suspicious death and required the attendance of a forensic pathologist. There was a considerable delay (forensic pathologists being few and sometimes having long distances to travel), but the pathologist also concluded, again after viewing the remains down the length of the garden, also by torchlight, that the Homicide Advisor (RT) should be called in. Upon arrival RT considered preserving the scene until daylight and calling a full forensic and major-incident team, but after a rapid examination of the area to assess the requirements needed, it became obvious that it was not a homicide case when he spotted several cloven hooves and part of a fresh sheepskin, part of a sheep's spinal column and a trail of blood, which in the poor light, resembled entrails. Further investigation revealed a sheep's head with readable identification tag on one ear.

It became apparent afterwards that someone had illegally acquired the sheep from which they had cut some joints of meat, then buried the rest and sold the house on without mentioning it to the new owners. Also, the cooling meat on the barbeque had attracted a scavenger (in the United Kingdom it is usually the fox, *Vulpes vulpes*) which had then become interested in the shallow burial and dug some of it up.

This apparently trivial story clearly illustrates some highly significant procedural flaws which might have had impact had the case truly been a forensic one. The attending officer made unfounded assumptions based on an inadequate reconnaissance of the scene and neglect of context (new house ownership, no evidence of the "corpse" during the barbeque, cooling meat to attract a scavenger). The pathologist also failed to examine the scene or remains. As stated above, the officer who first arrived at the "scene" should not necessarily be expected to be familiar with all the bones of all the possible animal carcasses which might be encountered; but should, however, either be able to identify a bone as non-human or be prepared to refer immediately to someone who can.

In this particular case, a more sensible approach could have been made from the start if only someone would have been prepared to get close enough to see the distinctive features of a sheep! Were a forensic anthropologist retained, the taking of a digital photograph that could then be forwarded by e-mail would have brought the officer close enough to view the animal remains clearly for what they actually were.

Ancient Burials

Archaeology is concerned with context; the position of finds (including human remains) and their relationship to each other and to the grave or other location. When bones are discovered accidentally, and the police are summoned to investigate, it is often assumed that the bones are ancient – or animal, as above – and they are therefore removed and taken to the anthropologist for confirmation of antiquity. Modern depositions can be fully skeletonised and those at the further end of the "forensic interest" time scale (decades rather than years) can be without odour, so there will be a few of these apparently ancient burials that are, in fact, of forensic interest. Removing the bones removes their context, which can be vital in establishing the identity of the victim and obtaining evidence.

We take this opportunity to recommend that a call to their local forensic anthropologist should precede any police interference at the scene however old the bones look (Ferllini, 2007). As above, unless it is obvious that she should attend the scene without delay, CD will often ask for digital photographs, from which she can examine the site and such features as the depth and form of the burial, or look at artefacts or contextual information which might establish the date of the deposition. These artefacts are sometimes seized and sent to the anthopologist (often with loose bones too) before consulting her, but although this is not optimal, it can still provide strong evidence for antiquity; for example, an Anglo-Saxon knife embedded in the pelvis of a skeleton, a Roman vase in the crook of the arm, and Bronze Age pottery fragments mingled with broken bones. Conversely, she might identify the remains as human and, from their condition, recent and requiring a full investigation (Duhig, 2003). Involving the local (non-forensic) archaeologist can also interfere with the investigation, for when the remains are recent, the forensic anthropologist will have to be called at that point, and time will be wasted in waiting, briefing and attempting to reconstruct the burial conditions and context of a now-disturbed grave.

We have described the anthropologists' role as being in two parts, that covering the archaeological (field/crime scene) and that of the osteological (mortuary/laboratory) functions. Due to the varied and ambiguous job titles and backgrounds of anthropologists and the poor training of scientific support and investigatory personnel, we find that one or other of these parts might be lost or misunderstood. For example, CD has on numerous occasions begun work at a crime scene and then been asked whether she knew an "anthropologist" who could examine the remains when she had excavated them; she has also been called directly to the mortuary by a pathologist colleague after the remains had been excavated by another forensic archaeologist (one whose expertise only extended to the crime-scene functions) or by the police themselves. This is inefficient at best. However, because of the various backgrounds from which forensic archaeologist and anthropologists come from, these situations do occur from time to time in the UK.

Case Study: A Recent Case of a Shallow Burial

A forensic archaeologist was called to recover fragmentary skeletal remains found shallowly buried in southern England. These were then taken to a forensic anthropologist who practised only the "anthropology" function. The anthropologist produced a profile of the individual, despite the absence of the skull and parts of the limbs, and the remains were identified as those of a missing young woman from London. While the anthropologist was on leave CD was asked to provide cover, and during that time a few other loose bones were brought which were compatible with those recorded from the missing woman. There was no cause of death, however, and it was felt to be imperative both to the investigation and for the bereaved family to locate the rest of the remains. Having a special interest in taphonomy (for discussions of the value of taphonomic interpretation see Haglund and Sorg, 1997a; Haglund and Sorg, 2002; especially Haglund and Sorg, 1997b; Scott and Connor, 1997; Dirkmaat and Adovasio, 1997; Ubelaker, 1997; Lyman, 2002; Reay, 2002; Hunter, 2002), CD made recommendations based on scavenger effects on body dispersal (Haglund and Sorg, 1997a; especially Haglund, 1997a;1997b; 1997c; Murrad, 1997) and from these the missing remains were found rapidly, the pathologist was able to make observations on potentially perimortem trauma and the family were able to have closure. The same result would have been achieved if normal search methods were used but speed and efficiency were added because CD as an osteologist knew what the missing body parts were and their size, shape, weight and transport potential, and as an archaeologist had knowledge of scavenger behaviour.

PROBLEM TWO: OVERSTAFFING AND ROLE OVERLAP

If the CSM, SIO or pathologist is sometimes ignorant of the existence of the anthropologist, or unaware that she can carry out investigation in both archaeology and physical anthropology, in many more situations the ignorance is only that pertaining to the specifics of their role. Unfortunately, these specific skills have some overlap with the expertise of other specialists who might be called to a crime scene or, to a lesser extent, to the mortuary, and the inexperienced manager who might not know who would be most suitable in a particular circumstance. Within a worst case scenario, every person on the major-incident staffing list will be called, "just in case," and apart from the impracticality at the crime scene, in criminal cases it gives more opportunities for defence lawyers to call upon these witnesses and confuse them before a jury. Fortunately, overstaffing is likely to be extremely rare in overseas deployments where financial and logistical constraints limit staff numbers. It is appropriate here, therefore, to outline the range of capacities which an archaeologist would be expected to possess.

Search

The archaeologist should have the basic archaeological field skills with which to discern an overall appreciation of the landscape and context of a possible burial site (e.g., Barker, 1982; Drewett, 1999; Killam, 2004); additionally, the archaeologist should interpret aerial photography (this can often be taken as a specialism within an archaeology degree) and be able to do map reading and drawing. By reading maps, the archaeologist can in turn look at the topography for potential access and burial feasibility. Knowledge of geology will also aid in interpretation of soil types for burial viability and their taphonomic effects on remains.

Moreover, a good understanding of the types, relative values and limitations of the geophysical prospecting techniques which can be applied, such as ground-penetrating radar or resistivity survey (see also Excavation: Body Recovery below) is desired; some archaeologists are specialists in the use of one or more of these techniques, although most call on the expertise of geophysical-prospection professionals when necessary (Pye and Croft, 2004).

Understanding of perpetrator behaviour is an advantage because the archaeologist spends much of her working life excavating, often ancient graves, and as such she has a better understanding than most of the factors involved in finding a suitable location for a grave and creating and re-filling it – and can imagine the difficulties, in the forensic context, of doing these things at speed and without detection.

The recording of flora and fauna, and interpretation of their relevance to the investigation, for example, plants of disturbed ground over graves, relevant faunas for disturbance and/or destruction of remains is a must for any archaeologist working a scene; however, once evidence needs to be properly processed and identified, a competent forensic botanist should be called in.

It can be seen that there is potential overlap with the expertise of the POLSA[4] and/or search team leader (general field craft, sometimes vegetation, combined with knowledge of patterns of perpetrator behaviour), air reconnaissance experts, dog handlers (field craft), geographers (maps and landscape), geologists (the same and soil science) and botanists. Further, there might be people involved in one or other of the geophysical techniques. Clearly, to invite all these persons, at the same time, to a scene would be unwieldy.

There is some guidance available apart from the SIO/CSM's own experience: the POLSA him or herself, the advisor from the National Crime and Operations Faculty (a central police resource) or the Forensic Search Advisory Group, a small conclave of police, forensic science personnel and freelance specialists who offer free advice on the most appropriate approaches and staffing for searches. In the US, Necro-Search International performs the same function on a considerably larger scale (France et al., 1992). All these organisations and individuals are invited, from time to time, to participate in long-term investigations

---

4. The term used in the UK for the Police Search Advisor, of whom every police force has at least one.

in areas such as the Balkans. As we have said, overstaffing is unlikely to be the case in international work, but it is to be hoped that senior investigators seek advice from these or similar experts or organisations in their home countries when they are tasked with staffing such missions. We have observed one nervous senior investigator, perhaps out of his professional depth, tending to the "just in case" approach mentioned above with detrimental results.

Case Study: Disorganisation in Central Asia

During the early part of 2000, a colleague of RT, a Scotland Yard Homicide Advisor, was assigned to an enquiry on the Pakistan/Afghanistan/Iran border region. Several years before, some military observers had been abducted and held hostage by one of the many militia groups within that area. Several months of intense but unsuccessful diplomatic negotiations were followed by news of their deaths/executions. During one of the many later sorties undertaken by Special Forces seeking out Al Qaeda suspects, several arrests were made and interrogations revealed the alleged sites of burial of the abducted military observers.

Upon the request of the country of origin of the missing observers, RT's colleague was flown to the region, accompanied by other senior detectives and a British Home Office forensic pathologist. Having met with the captors they discussed the planning, logistics and security aspects of identifying the graves and, potentially, recovering the victims. Despite the team's pleas for archaeological and anthropological assistance, the relevant authorities disallowed it. This was based on security grounds-personal safety of the civilian experts and the fact that their presence would increase the possibility of the incident being leaked to the press. The UK team cited the involvement of archaeological and anthropological experts in many UK criminal cases of political and personal sensitivity, with some also being involved in war crime investigations with the International Criminal Tribunals in Tanzania (for Rwanda – ICTR) and The Hague (for the former Yugoslavia – ICTY) with no such security breaches.

Ultimately, however, no such expertise was allowed and at the location the team spent many hours on several days, with their informant, attempting to locate the graves by guesswork and abortive digging, but with no result. The search was then called off but the team was resummoned a few months later to go through the same fruitless exercise again, albeit after having been assured that the informant had now recalled more detail of the grave positions and the military concerned had reconnoitered the scene and had narrowed down the search area.

This case exemplifies how the lack of intervention by a specialist in anthropology and archaeology hampered the effectiveness of the mission, hence resulting in the investigation being ultimately unsuccessful.

Excavation: Body Recovery

At the crime scene, there tend to be large numbers of staff-various investigators, scientific support personnel, the anthropologists, some of the specialists mentioned in the section above, additional ones such as entomologists and specialist advisors from the forensic science laboratories (e.g., in biological trace evidence, fibres and other materials), and the police logistics support. The latter topic will be addressed further on.

Archaeologists are very experienced in removing bodies or skeletons from the ground whilst obtaining maximum information from the grave cut, the fill and the artefacts[5] (based on standards such as Barker, 1982; Drewett, 1999; Hunter, et al., 1996). There are, however, a few police body-recovery teams who specialise in similar work. These teams are trained to remove the body from the grave with all relevant evidential material, and some — perhaps it has now become all — have received archaeological training to some level and can thus interpret depositional behaviour from the context of the grave. It might be superfluous to have an archaeologist if there is such a team attending. However, there are cases where inexperienced archaeologists and anthropologists are faced with rather complicated situations.

To illustrate, RT whilst working as a crime-scene co-ordinator for the British Forensic Team,[6] on one particular occasion organised the examination of a mass-murder site in western Kosova[7] in 1999. The team consisted of body-recovery police officers, scenes-of-crime officers (in

---

5. For non-archaeologists, these equate to: the dug boundary demarcating the human activity from the natural soil, sometimes conveniently preserving spade marks or shoe prints; the soil and other non-artefactual material returned to the grave; objects associated with the body, "exhibits" in forensic parlance.

6. Now, to some extent, replaced by the Centre for International Forensic Assistance(CIFA); Britain hosts another similar unit, InForce, while there are others in European countries (the work of some reflected in many of the chapters in this volume) in addition to the famous Argentine Forensic Anthropology Team and Physicians for Human Rights (PHR) based in the US.

7. The word Kosova is the preferred term among Kosovan-Albanians.

alternative terminology, crime-scene investigators), photographers, a pathologist, a mortuary technician and an anthropologist, accompanied by a military protection force. The site was a building in which 28 members of a Kosovan Albanian family had been machine-gunned, their bodies set alight with wood, tyres and other flammable material and eventually buried under the collapse of the building. The strategy adopted by RT was to grid the floor area and allocate a pair of staff members to each, sort and remove debris by hand to recover evidence and reveal the remains, and secondarily sift all debris away from the site as a double-check. A participating anthropologist with a limited amount of experience was initially uneasy with observing police officers carrying out this work, but was reassured when she found that small bones and teeth were being recovered (sometimes identified by their correct anatomical names by the police officers) along with cartridge casings and bullet heads. In eastern Kosova the following year, CD observed similar professionalism by police body-recovery teams.

It must be said, however, that although the investigator will set the parameters for the body recovery and often all that is required is that the human remains and exhibits are obtained, in a situation where detailed excavation, interpretation of stratigraphy (the sequence of soil layers and their disturbance) and delicate exposure and clearance of fugitive grave-cut edges is needed, the forensic archaeologist is essential. Large mass graves and extended operations require field archaeologists with considerable relevant field experience, obtained in previous human-rights investigations and/or complex urban archaeology (for example see Chapters 9 and 11 of this volume; Hunter and Cox, 2005).

Identification and Other Mortuary Roles

There is less opportunity for overstaffing in the mortuary, at home or abroad, where at a minimum there is likely to be a pathologist, mortuary technician, anthropologist and at least one exhibits officer, who may act additionally as a photographer, with the senior investigator, his deputy and/or other detectives − depending on the complexity of the case − keeping out of the way. Some of these staff might be duplicated, for example, more scientific support staff. In the UK there might be a representative of the Coroner, and there could also be a forensic odontologist, a fingerprints officer and a facial artist. At this stage, there is the opportunity for crowding and interfering with each others' types of evidence and the sequence in which it should be recovered. The U.S. Disaster Mortuary Operational Response Teams (DMORTs) list 20 specialist skills which can be made available to assist at mass disasters (DMORT 2006), and although DMORTs are not deployed in the context of human rights issues, the list gives an indication of the quantity of personnel potentially working on a case.

All of the interventions described above are subject to more than merely overstaffing, however. Demarcation difficulties can easily descend into dispute; there may be many highly-qualified people involved, all (one hopes) with great confidence in their expertise, and some with the belief that their particular speciality will make the most significant contribution to the investigation. These will occasionally include academics who perhaps carry out forensic work rarely, and have a mind-set geared to leisurely university schedules with the opportunity to research questions of interest as they occur. Some staff will have some knowledge of each others' disciplines, but they might not have enough to understand the scope or constraints of each, and − let it be said − some, in our experience, can treat the needs of their colleagues and the investigation in a way which is cavalier at best and objectionable and unprofessional at worst (also see Chapter 7 of this volume). Exacerbating this can be xenophobia, not only of colleagues from different countries but from different backgrounds and training, and, sadly to say, we have observed a very small amount of both racist and sexist behaviour.[8]

We offer, however, a happy example here. It is relatively unusual for us to find that forensic artists have been called, but their use is, fortunately for the progress of human identification, becoming more frequent. CD worked with an artist who wished to sketch the skull of a burned body after the facial skin had been flayed during the autopsy (note that it would have been preferable for the face to have been sketched, however changed by burning, before this flaying and the subsequent shrinkage and distortion of the skin, and this is to be recommended in future cases). The artist asked CD to discuss with her the possible ethnic affiliation of the individual, his body build and facial proportions, and the effects of burning on the shape of some of the features. This was a profitable collaboration, enhanced by a discussion with

---

8. Not in the police but in other specialists. The police are sometimes accused of one "institutional-ism" or other but they would at least have the excuse of being a closed society, which the outside consultants do not.

the odontologist on some unusual dental features which also agreed with possible ethnic attributions. It can be seen that professional arrogance could have intruded, even interfered with the identification process, were the artist to have regarded her rare skills as of more significance than the others.

Case Study: A Terrorist Attack in Sri Lanka

In early 1993 RT, two senior Scotland Yard detectives and a UK Home Office forensic pathologist were invited by the Sri Lankan government to assist with the investigations of several political assassinations, shootings and bombings in Colombo, thought to have been perpetrated by the Tamil Tigers, possibly in conjunction with other terrorist groups with political agendas. RT was also asked to assist with forensic training for the Sri Lankan police service. Over the following few weeks, the group travelled around sectors of the country that were under government control, but just prior to the May Day holiday they were instructed by the British Embassy to remove themselves, under the supervision of a Sri Lankan protection team, to a remote part of the country for their own safety. The then President of Sri Lanka, Ranasinghe Premadasa, would be addressing and passing amongst the crowds in the main square in Colombo on May 1st and this greatly heightened the possibility of an attempted terrorist attack.

On that particular day, a bomb was set off in the Colombo main square: the President and approximately 26 to 28 of his guards were killed and a multitude of innocent bystanders maimed and injured. The attack succeeded due to inadequate security precautions: Premadasa's personal valet and a "friend" (probably Tamil Tiger "sleepers") entered the inner security cordon, pushing a pedal cycle, without any body searches taking place, and detonated a body bomb connected to explosives in the pedal cycle once they got close enough to speak with the President. The Sri Lankan authorities asked the team to return immediately to Colombo to assist with the ensuing enquiry, but because their return would be delayed because of safety and transport issues resulting from the state of emergency, RT gave telephone instructions regarding crime-scene security and the requirement for mortuary facilities, to which the entire Sri Lankan Scenes of Crime Unit at police HQ was assigned.

Upon arrival at the location of the bombing, however, it was found that everything had been removed; all that remained was the crime scene cordon tape protecting an empty space, within which was a small quantity of debris, visible damage to a few buildings, and a dried area where a heavy volume of blood had been spilt. All the victims and body parts had been removed on a military truck to the public mortuary, where RT and the pathologist found a mound of bodies and body parts in the yard, covered by tarpaulins and similar materials and "identified" by outer clothing and insignia of military and police uniforms – valueless given that virtually all the deceased, apart from the President and a few aides, wore senior military or police uniforms. A wrist watch worn by the President on that day (inscribed as a recent gift from his wife) was the main point of his identification, and RT recalls vividly a senior police officer holding the severed head of either the "friend" or the valet towards the television camera, and asking if anyone could identify the individual.

The request for forensic anthropological expertise was refused, apparently partly due to the political sensitivity of the incident, as the authorities did not want anyone outside government circles to witness the current condition of the deceased and be aware of the state of the criminal investigation. Further, the government pathologists felt that they were more than capable of carrying out the task of identifying the bodies. The severed head was subsequently identified as being that of the valet and RT travelled later to his village, accompanied by the police Scenes of Crime team and large, heavily-armed protection squads, in order to carry out a forensic search of his living quarters. It transpired that this search did reveal evidence of use to the Sri Lankan authorities. Shortly afterwards, the UK Foreign Office instructed the team to leave the country.

This case illustrates the difficulties experienced on a practical basis by international forensic teams, including the negative consequences of a poorly-managed crime scene and institutional unwillingness to accept the intervention of an anthropologist, resulting from both local preconceptions and political interference.

Case Study: Identification and Discovery of Covert Graves

In Kosova during 1999, and again in 2000, the British Forensic Team (BFT) participated in hundreds of similar but intrinsically different body recoveries. In some instances, the team had to operate within legitimate cemeteries where victims of genocide and mass murder had been concealed by their killers within legitimate burials. Separating the legitimate from the illegitimate graves required stringent exhumation procedures and the combination of anthropological and pathological assessments. If a family disbelieved the authorities' assertion that their loved one had died naturally in hospital, this could be verified by an independent body – hence the intervention of the BFT. If the on-site anthropologist had access to medical records from a nearby hospital, it was possible to undertake the task at the grave side, and in the absence of any records, but with the correct expertise on tap, an adequate analysis could be achieved and the death eliminated or added to the BFT remit.

In one instance, a female victim had reportedly been shot by a sniper and had been removed by friends to a local hospital. Treatment was unsuccessful and she later died. This could be confirmed because of the obvious evidence of surgical incisions and remedial surgery present upon the body, details which also assisted in the positive identification of the victim. In another case, a totally skeletonised body was being recovered by an anthropologist and a body-recovery colleague was sieving the bottom of the grave for small bones and fragments of the smashed cranium (death was by means of a close-contact gunshot wound to the head). It was found that the grave was constructed directly above another, unrecorded, grave which was consequently excavated. As a result, another victim with a similar fatal head wound was discovered.

This type of situation was a recurring theme from time to time in Kosova. By contrast with the previous case study, such victims might not have been recovered or identified had the expertise of an anthropologist not been available in the field, with countless hours of unnecessary and arduous work being saved.

PROBLEM THREE: HUMAN RESOURCES MANAGEMENT

The above has now introduced us to a third source of difficulty, that of the need for highly informed and sensitive management of a large number of people from disparate backgrounds, some of whom come with problematic personality traits. If this is important in our home countries, examining, shall we say, a single clandestine grave and its unidentified occupant, how much more important it is in a country not our own, examining a mass grave and its several, hundreds or thousands of occupants. We offer a few straightforward recommendations.

Staff Management

Except in emergencies, it will always prove more efficient in the long run to delay commencement of work – whether search, excavation or autopsy – until there has been sufficient planning involving discussions with all involved and assessment by the CSM or SIO of the needs of each. If this seems painfully obvious, we have to stress that we have seen precipitate commencement lead to inefficient investigation. The most common fault is a tendency to put in specialists in an incorrect sequence during the search:

1. Using a search team at the beginning of the evaluation of an area introduces a large number of (probably heavy) feet that can damage the human remains or other evidential material beneath and trample animal tracks or droppings before a faunal specialist has had the opportunity to examine them – compare the care that would be taken to record footprints or tyre tracks before they had to be walked over.
2. Stripping an area of its vegetation before the archaeologist/anthropologist or botanist has had access removes some of the evidence of ruderal vs. climax plant communities and length of growth period.
3. Bones are not to be collected and taken to the anthropologist, even if they appear to be ancient, irrelevant to the investigation or already disturbed. Their simple disturbance, itself being a taphonomic factor, can be informative and context is vital to interpretation (Ferllini, 2007).

During the excavation we recommend:

1. In order to avoid the problem of too many people overall, a senior investigator, well-versed in the disciplines of his specialists can assess who will be needed and who can reasonably be left out in that specific case. An honourable specialist will admit when they are not needed at a site because they cannot make much of a positive contribution at that stage, or because their role overlaps with another, essential, specialist.

2. Too many people close to the grave site creates an increased potential for contamination and damage to the scene and the human remains. For single graves, we recommend an inner cordon within which it would be usual to find no more than the anthropologist and two other people (anthropologist's assistants or scenes-of-crime officers) with their equipment, plus a photographer if not covered by one of these three. The exhibits officer should remain outside this cordon if close enough for exhibits to be passed directly; even the CSM rarely needs to be inside. There should be little or no need for an SIO, although sometimes their enthusiasm can overcome their prudence. We have heard of an SIO walking in the victim's pooled blood and tracking bloody footprints up the stairs in his eagerness to see the scene.

3. In cramped conditions, there may be too many people on top of the body. In an international investigation CD, newly arrived on deployment, found herself in the first single grave with the body recovery team of three and the mortuary technician (awaiting the first body and therefore helping to recover it). A request to RT to reduce numbers was immediately responded to.

4. Speed of investigation: forensic examinations of scenes may take many hours, yet SIOs and CSMs are sometimes anxious (even aggravated) by the length of time a forensic-archaeology activity requires, and it requires a strong nerve on the part of the anthropologist to keep to the excavation plan and time scale. There is a need for awareness from the CSM that archaeology is a complicated combination of outdoor activity, doing dirty and heavy "earth-moving" work, and highly detailed forensic work requiring accuracy and attention to protocols.

Concerning mortuary work, as we have illustrated, there are rarely too many people in the mortuary. There are, however, occasions when there are too many people around or in the body. All the staff might be crowded at the table or gurney and sometimes several pairs of hands could be working on defleshing, removal of organs, examination of teeth and so on. All these people, however, well-gowned and masked, have the potential to contaminate the body or to intrude on each others' areas, and this is particularly likely to occur on an international mission when pressure of work requires all specialists to complete their particular tasks at high speed. CD has experienced situations in which she has been obliged to step away from the body because the jostling of a large number of staff prevented efficient working.

Safety

The matter of attention to safety can be tiresome, but essential. With archaeology being an "outdoorsy" discipline, practitioners often have an ethos of disregard, indeed disdain, for health and safety procedures. In one actual incident during a mission, a newly-arrived anthropologist, in her eagerness to see the remains, leaped down into an opened grave and was struck on the head and bowled over by the JCB (back-hoe) bucket; and CD had a narrow escape from the same accident. Apart from the obvious need for restraint from the individual, this calls for robust management by the CSM who may become unpopular when insisting upon the wearing of hard hats and ensuring a watcher is positioned with a warning whistle or similar implement to draw attention to possible danger.

Within the mortuary we have heard of very few occasions of injury, despite the hazards of sharp instruments, and few other safety breaches. This is probably due to the discipline imposed by mortuary managers and technicians, although in a lengthy autopsy surgical gloves begin to slip slightly on sweaty hands, dissection knives become greasy, attention begins to wander due to fatigue and there is increased potential for injury.[9] In one instance, a highly-disrupted body, judicially exhumed for reinvestigation, required two pathologists, an anthropologist and her assistant, the mortuary technician and a photographer, of whom four were wielding dissection knives or scalpels. When mortuaries are informal and contingent, as in international investigations – sometimes being no more than a blow-up tent or some tables outdoors – there is more potential for hazards. Again, safety measures taken by the individual are essential (the anthropologist on an international placement who cut up her lunch with a surgical knife deserves the reprimand and opprobrium she received for her disregard of safety and the protocols of an investigation) but they must also be imposed from above by the senior investigator.

---

9. For example, CD finds that standard surgical gloves are rarely small enough for her, and therefore they have a greater tendency to slip. She recommends everyone should carry several pairs of latex or nitrile gloves, according to requirements, that fit properly, and that suitable gloves should be sourced if working abroad.

CONCLUSIONS

We believe that training for all concerned in forensic investigations should be as comprehensive as possible, to inform the investigator and the specialists about each others' work, to introduce them to each other in situations away from the crucial one of the crime scene, and to keep dialogue going through conferences and publications.

We emphasise the necessity for timely and forthright discussion at the initial planning conference, in the field and at updates, behaviour denoting mutual respect between professionals and the integration of the anthropologist within a clear command structure. In addition to all other responsibilities, the Crime Scene Manager is obliged to undertake human resources management at the scene, balancing the requirements of each team member or unit, taking into account their needs for access, timing and resources against their potential contribution to the investigation, and integrating the involvement of each into the overall strategy. This requires him/her to manage personnel from widely different disciplines who might be inclined to treat each other with suspicion and who might be somewhat inflexible. He also needs to deal with practical issues deriving from the HR function, including such aspects as health and safety, which might be little regarded by some of his staff.

For the anthropologist – or, indeed, any other visiting specialist – the rules must be, as a minimum for harmonious and effective working: No Academics (must adapt to the pace and requirements of forensic cases), No Prima Donnas (there must be respect and co-ordination with colleagues) and No Clowns (must not disregard health and safety issues).

REFERENCES

Barker, P. (1982). *Techniques of archaeological excavation.* London: Batsford.

Brickley, M., and Ferllini, R. (2007). Forensic anthropology: Development in two continents. In *Forensic anthropology: Case studies from Europe*, Brickley, M. and Ferllini, R. (Eds.). Springfield: Charles C Thomas. In press.

Dirkmaat, D.C., and Adovasio, J.M. (1997). The role of archaeology in the recovery and interpretation of human remains from an outdoor forensic setting. In *Forensic taphonomy: The postmortem fate of human remains*, Haglund, W.D. and Sorg, M.H. (Eds.). Boca Raton: CRC Press, pp. 39–64.

Disaster Mortuary Operational Response Teams (DMORTs) (2006). http://www.dmort.org

Drewett, P.L. (1999). *Field archaeology: An introduction.* London: UCL Press.

Duhig, C. (2003). Non-forensic remains: The use of forensic archaeology, anthropology and burial taphonomy. *Science and Justice, 43*(4):211–214.

Ferllini, R. (2007). Bone scatter on chalk: The importance of osteological knowledge and environmental assessment. In *Forensic anthropology: Case studies from Europe*, Brickley, M., and Ferllini, R. Springfield: Charles C Thomas. In press.

France, D.L., Griffin, T.J., Swanburg, J.G., Lindemann, J.W., Davenport, G.C., Trammell, V., Travis, C.T., Kondratieff, B., Nelson, A., Castellano, K., Hopkins, D., and Adair, T. (1992). A multidisciplinary approach to the detection of clandestine graves. *J. Forensic Sciences, 37*(6):1445–1458.

Haglund, W.D. (1997a). Dogs and coyotes: Postmortem involvement with human remains. In *Forensic taphonomy: The postmortem fate of human remains*, Haglund, W.D., and Sorg, M.H. (Eds.). Boca Raton: CRC Press, pp. 367–381.

Haglund, W.D. (1997b). Scattered skeletal human remains: Search strategy considerations for locating missing teeth. In *Forensic taphonomy: The postmortem fate of human remains*, Haglund, W.D., and Sorg, M.H. (Eds.). Boca Raton: CRC Press, pp. 383–394.

Haglund, W.D. (1997c). Rodents and human remains. In *Forensic taphonomy: The postmortem fate of human remains*, Haglund, W.D., and Sorg, M.H. (Eds.). Boca Raton: CRC Press, pp. 405–414.

Haglund, W.D., and Sorg, M.H. (Eds.). (1997a). *Forensic taphonomy: The postmortem fate of human remains*. Boca Raton: CRC Press.

Haglund, W.D., and Sorg, M.H. (Eds.). (1997b). Method and theory of forensic taphonomy research. In *Forensic taphonomy: The postmortem fate of human remains*. Boca Raton: CRC Press, pp. 13–26.

Haglund, W.D., and Sorg, M.H. (Eds.). (2002). *Advances in forensic taphonomy: Method, theory and archaeological perspectives*. Boca Raton: CRC Press.

Hunter, J. (2002). Foreword: A pilgrim in forensic archaeology – A personal view. In *Advances in forensic taphonomy: Method, theory, and archaeological perspectives*, Haglund, W.D., and Sorg, M.H. (Eds.). Boca Raton: CRC Press, pp. xxv– xxxii.

Hunter, J., and Cox, M. (2005). *Forensic archaeology: Advances in theory and practice*. London: Routledge.

Hunter, J., Roberts, C., and Martin, A. (1996). *Studies in crime: An introduction to forensic archaeology*. London: Batsford.

Killam, E.W. (2004). *The detection of human remains*. Springfield: Charles C Thomas, Ltd.

Lyman, R.L. (2002). Foreword. In *Advances in forensic taphonomy: Method, theory, and archaeological perspectives*, Haglund, W.D., and Sorg, M.H. (Eds.). Boca Raton: CRC Press, pp. xix–xxi.

Murrad, , T.A. (1997). The utilization of faunal evidence in the recovery of human remains. In *Forensic taphonomy: The postmortem fate of human remains*, Haglund, W.D., and Sorg, M.H. (Eds.). Boca Raton: CRC Press, pp. 395–404.

Pepper, I.A. (2005). *Crime scene investigation: Methods and procedures*. Maidenhead: Open University Press.

Pye, K., and Croft, D.J. (2004). *Forensic geoscience: Principles, techniques and applications*. London: Geological Society.

Reay, D.T. (2002). Foreword. In *Advances in forensic taphonomy: Method, theory, and ar-

chaeological perspectives, Haglund, W.D., and Sorg, M.H. (Eds.). Boca Raton: CRC Press, pp. xxiii–xxiv.

Scott, D.D. and Connor, M. (1997). Context delicti: Archeological context in forensic work. In *Forensic taphonomy: The postmortem fate of human remains.* Boca Raton: CRC Press, pp. 27–38.

Ubelaker, D.H. (1997). Taphonomic applications in forensic anthropology. In *Forensic taphonomy: The postmortem fate of human remains.* Boca Raton: CRC Press, pp. 77–90.

Chapter 5

ARCHAEOLOGY AND THE FORENSIC PATHOLOGIST

PETER ELLIS

INTRODUCTION

Forensic pathology is the study of disease and injury in the context of a legal investigation. Therefore, the role of the forensic pathologist is to examine human remains so as to satisfy the requirements of the legal framework under which the analysis is being undertaken. This may be a small domestic investigation, whereby the death of a single person has been uncovered, or it may be a major international program to study the deaths of huge numbers of people in incidents of genocide or war crimes. The forensic pathologist has a responsibility to determine the identity of the decedent(s), the cause of death and, if possible, the circumstances surrounding and the manner of death.

The interaction between the forensic archaeologist and the pathologist centres on the information and knowledge that can be uncovered at the site of burial. It is the utilisation of that information that allows the pathologist to understand much of the evidence relevant to the interment. The recovery of the remains is the first step in the pathology process that leads ultimately to the determination of identity. Additionally, in the establishment of the cause of death, the state of the body at burial, and the presence of location evidence, may prove to be crucial factors in completing the pathological investigation. It is archaeological expertise which provides that early evidence. Often the circumstances and manner of death can only be determined after proper exhumation, as the method of burial may itself provide essential evidence to support

101

a particular contention. It is in this way that archaeology and pathology interrelate and coexist.

WHAT IS FORENSIC PATHOLOGY?

Pathology is the study of disease and injury, including its causation and diagnosis, and the understanding of the progression of that disease in both the living and the dead. Forensic pathology is the study and practice of pathology when conducted in a legal framework. So the application of that study to a medicolegal context warrants the consideration of a whole range of issues that would not necessarily concern the practising clinical pathologist. For example, the very involvement of the pathologist in the clinical management of a patient is usually initiated either by the patient himself, or more usually, by the patient's medical attendant. Implicit in this involvement is the consent of the patient to have certain tests performed, or procedures conducted. Sometimes this consent needs to be formalised in a signed document, but more frequently, the very presence of the patient in the pathologist's laboratory implies consent, and provides the necessary legal framework for the conducting of the testing.

As forensic pathology must be accomplished with legal processes in mind, the application of all aspects of the investigation should only be attempted when the correct legal authorisations have been obtained. In practical terms, this will vary enormously with the nature of the situation, and the circumstances in which the investigation is to be conducted. For example, the possible exhumation of a murder victim from land that is private property may require the provision of a search warrant from the relevant authorities. Failure to obtain such legal authorisation may render any evidence subsequently recovered unusable in legal proceedings, even if that evidence is incontrovertible and probative. The forensic pathologist, usually employed in some form of public capacity, is always mindful of the need to legitimise his/her findings by placing them in the correct medicolegal context. This context needs to be considered with reference to the particular country in which the investigation is being conducted. Therefore, it is appropriate that when archaeological investigation is to be utilised or attempted in any individual case, the pathologist should be consulted at an early stage, so as to ensure that any evidence collected will be possible in the following legal proceedings. The legal proceedings may be a murder trial, a civil hearing, an international war crimes tribunal, or even just an enquiry where no individual has been indicted or charged. Nevertheless, it is incumbent on all investigators to ensure that the evidence is collected in a manner so as to fulfill all the necessary requirements of the legal jurisdiction in which the hearing is being conducted.

The majority of investigations are carried out in domestic policing situations, where the location and recovery of a single or small number of bodies is the only focus. In that situation, the needs of the local jurisdiction must be met in full, and this may involve the aforementioned search warrants, local authority approvals, clearance from public utilities, and agreements from local interest groups. It is appropriate that as the pathologist will probably be presenting his findings in a subsequent legal forum then he should note all the authorities received and record them in the report that he will inevitably prepare. In that way, all the findings can be viewed and assessed on merit, and not in the context of potential legal challenge. In those situations where the excavation or exhumation is to be conducted on a possible mass grave, then the authorities are usually different. Such investigations are often carried out in areas of current or previous conflict, and the legal administration may not be as well developed. Nevertheless, it is proper for correct authority to be sought before any investigation is undertaken.

HOW DOES FORENSIC PATHOLOGY OPERATE?

The forensic pathologist is a medical practitioner. The training and experience of forensic pathologists vary significantly between countries and this may be reflected in the emphasis that individuals place on different aspects of their practice. For example, in some countries the forensic pathologist is trained in pathology but also practices clinical forensic medicine. That is to say the performance of autopsies is but a small part of the daily routine. Clinical forensic medicine, or the examination of patients who have been possible victims of some kind of assault, is an extremely important specialty, but its practitioner needs different skills to the pathologist who diagnoses injury or disease by anatomical dissection. Having said that, the methodology of forensic pathology practice is not very different from clinical medicine.

The clinician, when approached by a patient with some ailment, conducts the investigation with the aim to establish what pathological process is affecting that patient at that time. Once that diagnosis is made, then the pathological condition can be appropriately treated. The investigation follows a well-recognised pattern, whereby the doctor gets information from the patient by taking the history, and then conducts a physical examination. At this stage, there is likely to be a single diagnosis or at least a list of possible differential diagnoses that the doctor considers. Further analysis using other technologies such as biopsy, radiology or laboratory testing will usually confirm the specific pathological process that is affecting the patient at that time. The patient can then be appropriately treated. The forensic pathologist undergoes the same general investigative processes, but the focus is a little different. The history is still taken but, as the "patient" is usually deceased, that information must be obtained from a different source. That is usually the police, medical attendants, family members, or even witnesses. Once that history is obtained, then the physical examination is conducted. That, of course, is the autopsy, and once that is completed (possibly with ancillary investigations such as toxicology, histology, microbiology or anthropology) then a diagnosis is, hopefully, made, but this diagnosis is not of the pathological process currently active in the patient. It is, in fact, a diagnosis of the event or events that culminated in the death of the "patient." Therefore, it is the aim of the forensic pathological investigation to recreate the event or series of events that conclude with the death. All the observations made by the pathologist, or any of the ancillary investigators are combined to formulate this story that explains how the person came to be deceased, and possibly how the body came to be in the location or situation in which it is found. The collection of all evidence in the investigation, including that of an archaeological nature, must be geared to development of this chronicle of the events leading to death.

Since it is frequently the principal responsibility of the pathologist to gather together the evidence needed to allow authorities to finalise all the investigations, and to reach conclusions regarding the death(s), he must be satisfied that each part of the investigation has been professionally and comprehensively completed. It is necessary, then, to consider the various parts of the pathologist's responsibilities, and discuss how archaeology contributes to their successful completion.

The pathologist endeavours to determine or investigate a number of different aspects of a death, or deaths. Specifically, he may be required to offer opinion or assist in the investigation into the following:

a. The identity of the deceased,
b. The time or date of death,
c. The place of death (or at least whether that was the same as the place of discovery),
d. The cause of death,
e. The manner or mode of death,
f. The presence of disease or injury that may or may not have contributed to death, or to the circumstances culminating in death.

This long list of tasks is, of course, not performed in isolation. Indeed, it is mandatory to recognise that all aspects of this investigation need to be conducted using a team approach. Each stage of the process utilises a multi-disciplinary group of investigators. While most laypersons recognise the pathologist's role within the autopsy room, apart from the occasional depiction in popular television, most people would not realise that the autopsy commences well before the body reaches the morgue. So it is often necessary for the pathologist to commence the investigation at the place where the body is discovered.

Identity Of The Deceased

Establishing the identity of the dead is an essential part, and often the first part, of the postmortem investigation. Notwithstanding the statutory requirement of the authorising coroner or magistrate, there are a number of reasons why identification is so important:

1. To commence and facilitate police enquiries. The identity of the victim(s) is an integral and vital part of the early stages of any death investigation.
2. To provide information for and closure to relatives. This is a basic humanitarian need.
3. To satisfy various legal requirements with respect to estates, property, insurance protocols.
4. To confirm that death has occurred, so as to satisfy official and statistical needs.

5. To facilitate appropriate disposal of a particular body by burial or cremation.

Identification

Visual identification, where the external appearance of the body is viewed by a close relative or friend, who then indicates whether the appearances are those of the presumed deceased person, is often regarded as the standard by which other methods of identification should be judged. Even when the body has not deteriorated as a result of decomposition, this process is flawed, and should be supported by some objective assessment of identity. While many bodies exhumed with the aid of forensic archaeology will be decomposed, for reasons outlined above, archaeological techniques can also be used to uncover recently dug graves. So in some cases, despite the involvement of an archaeologist, the remains are preserved well enough for some investigators to consider using visual identification as a primary means of confirming identity. This is usually inappropriate, and may result in incorrect identification and misdirection of the investigation. Reasons why visual identification is often flawed include:

- Facial features in the dead are often altered from their living state. There may be a loss or change in colour, the skin turgor is altered, and the shape may appear different because the body is observed lying rather than the more usual vertical position.
- The face is visualised without the usual adornments (jewellery, spectacles, makeup).
- The identifying person is often stressed, and therefore not necessarily concentrating optimally.
- There may be injuries, blood, effects of burning and decomposition.
- The surrounding facilities are rarely conducive to stress-free viewing.
- There may even be a subtle, albeit unintended, pressure to make the identification.

Therefore, objective methods are required to complete the identification process, especially when the remains show even early stages of postmortem deterioration. Identification of a decomposed body can be affected using any of a number of different markers. Those that are unique to any individual, such as the DNA profile, fingerprint pattern and dental comparison are said to be **primary identifiers**. Other techniques such as examination of clothing, personal effects, medical and radiological features, physical attributes, and scars or tattoos are said to be secondary identifiers. The **secondary identifiers** should only be used in conjunction with one or more of the other identifying methods before the identification is confirmed. On the other hand, if primary identifiers are available, then they may be sufficient to confirm the identity without resort to any other method.

The forensic archaeologist must be mindful of the need to collect evidence to facilitate identification, whether the case is a single recent murder being exhumed from a clandestine grave (known in Australia as "bush burials") or whether it is part of a major excavation of a mass interment from a scene of older international conflict. Long after the International Criminal Tribunal of the former Yugoslavia (ICTY) finished collecting evidence for its various prosecutions of indicted suspected war criminals, the process of identifying victims of the various atrocities, such as the Srebrenica massacre, is continuing. Of course, in these cases, the remains are likely to be wholly skeletonised, and anthropological techniques may be needed to identify specific abnormalities that may allow recognition of individual features. As the remains may well be commingled in a mass grave situation, skilful archaeological methods are essential when removing individuals from such sites.

Primary Identifiers

The DNA profile of every individual is unique (excepting identical siblings) and so DNA profiling of human remains is an obvious technique that will allow identification (Rudin and Inman, 2002). As it would be impractical (and unnecessary) to sequence the entire DNA of all samples, the simpler technique of comparing only parts of the DNA with those of family members is perfectly adequate to conclude that an individual is almost certain to be a close relative. While the majority of the genetic material in the human genome resides in the nucleus of the cell (nuclear DNA) some additional material does exist in cell organelles. Of these, the most important are the mitochondria. Mitochondrial DNA (mtDNA) differs from nuclear DNA in a number of ways. It is often abundant in any cell, and is fairly small, so it is rather resistant to degradation, and consequently, it is often the DNA of choice in badly decomposed bodies, especially those in which skeletonisation has been completed, or is nearing final stages. However, unlike nuclear DNA, which is inherited from both parents, mtDNA has lineage through the maternal line. Therefore, it may only be possible to identify the vertical lineage, but not its horizontal equivalent. The family can be identified, but it is not necessarily possible to distinguish an individual from within a set of siblings. The exhumation must be performed with the possibility of the collection of suitable DNA in mind.

Fingerprints can only be of value in the non-skeletonised body, but it is perhaps surprising how effective fingerprinting can be with a cadaver showing advanced putrefaction. As long as some ridge pattern remains, even if confined to the palms or soles, it may be possible to record it in a form that can be usefully applied to comparison with a previous record, or with latent prints from some possession of the presumed person. So the removal of the body from the site of interment must be conducted in such a manner that any fingerprints can be preserved, and subsequently examined.

Dental examination, including dental charting, x-ray and comparison with antemortem dental records, is beyond the scope of this chapter; however, especially in contemporary exhumations, and in western countries (where dental charting is usual) the removal of the body from the grave must be carried out while ensuring the preservation of any dentition that may be present. Teeth are very resilient, and even those teeth that drop out after death during the decomposition process, and during the rough handling of burial, must be retrieved and saved for the odontologist. The need to have antemortem dental records means that often this identification method may not prove to be of use to the odontologist. In many countries dentists are not familiar with the value of charting, or do not have the time or resources to conduct it routinely. So each case and situation must be considered on its own merits. The examination of specialist x-rays, such as orthopantomograms (OPGs) and their comparison with antemortem records, will facilitate dental identification. Occasionally, it may be possible to superimpose such antemortem x-rays with special photographs of the exhumed skull, and confirm identification by matching the exact placement of teeth, gaps, defects and even sinus patterns.

Secondary Identifiers

Clothing and personal effects are often used to aid in the identification process. While many exhumed remains are skeletonised, it is not uncommon that if the victims were murdered while clothed, then those clothes remain, albeit in a damaged condition (Fig. 5-1). Therefore it may be possible to allow someone familiar with the clothing of the deceased to identify items which they recognise. The possibility that clothing may be similar, or may have been replaced or exchanged, means that this method should not be used as a primary identifier, but it may allow narrowing of the search pattern when selecting cases for DNA or dental comparison.

Personal effects, such as documents, may be quite specific and are often used as the sole identifier. It must be admitted, however, that this too may be falsified in that documents are easily switched and, like clothing, should be used to reduce the search pattern for one of the primary identifiers.

Physical, medical and radiological features can be loosely classified into those features that normally characterise the individual, and those that are abnormal, but are specific for a particular person. The former are those attributes such as race, sex, stature and age. With skeletal remains,

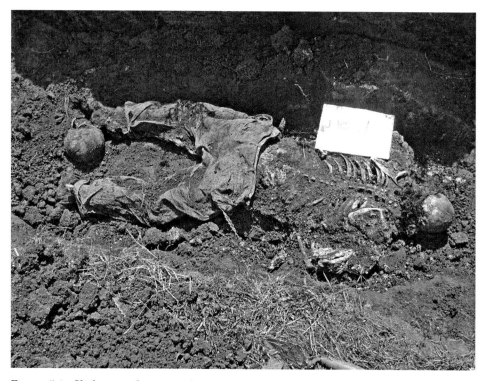

Figure 5-1. Skeletonised remains lying face down in a grave in Pristina, Kosovo. Note a second skull near the feet at the left of the photo and the remaining clothing.

these may be determined with a fair degree of accuracy by anthropological examination of various bones or groups of bones. This determines the need for careful exhumation, and in particular when the presence of multiple victims in a single grave site means that there may be commingling of the remains. Initially, this anthropological study can indicate either how many victims are present, or at least the minimum number of individuals (MNI). Individual remains may be examined to determine racial origin, especially when the skull is present. It is sometimes possible to racially classify remains into one of the main groups (Caucasian, Mongoloid or Black) but frequently, there may have been some racial intermingling or the racial grouping may not fall into one of the defined classes. In the recent conflict in the Solomon Islands in the southwest Pacific between 1999 and 2003, there were a number of racial sets that originated from various island groups. Fighting between islanders from Malaita and those originating in Guadalcanal has resulted in many deaths and multiple burial grounds. Careful anthropological examination at the grave site in such a situation may assist in placing the remains within one of the defined groups. There are two ethnic groups, the Istabu from Guadalcanal and the Malaitans from Malaita. As both groups are of Melanesian origin, this distinction has largely been done by comparison of artefacts. This permits furthering of the investigation of the activity that culminated in the death of the victims being exhumed. The description of the detailed examination of remains with the purpose of determining sex, age and stature belongs elsewhere, but suffice it to say that it is an essential part of the initial examination of exhumed remains (topic discussed in Chapter 6 of this volume). The archaeologist, through careful uncovering and retrieval of the remains, initiates this process. The forensic pathologist is required, if possible, to identify the body as part of his autopsy, and information made available to him by a professional archaeological examination at the time of disinterment will be invaluable in aiding the identification process.

The presence of evidence of medical conditions, previous medical procedures, and even prosthetic devices, is invaluable to the pathologist attempting to identify the victims of mass interment, as well as of single homicide. Skin survives surprisingly well in some burial conditions, and careful examination at an early stage allows the observation of scars, tattoos and other surface abnormalities that may facilitate identification. It behoves the archaeologist to pay special attention to the preservation and careful treatment of the skin during excavation when it seems likely that skin remains, even if it has deteriorated with time and soil conditions. Tattoos are surprisingly resilient and as the pigment is often present in quite deep layers of the skin, even the loss of the surface (a common result of early decomposition) may not render the tattoo image unrecognisable. Additionally, scars are often deep structures and very prominent, especially in some races where skin thickening or keloid may be common.

Skeletal abnormalities that are peculiar to an individual may be enough to allow identification to proceed to the primary identifier state. An example of an abnormal skeletal feature found during examination of bones exhumed in Kosovo is illustrated in Figure 5-2. The use of x-rays to demonstrate skeletal abnormalities may sometimes facilitate this identification, and the use of this technology should be included in any forward planning of the excavation and subsequent examination. Discrete abnormalities, such as healing fractures, metal prostheses, pacemakers, bone disease, or congenital defects are definite aids in establishing identity. They may be damaged by careless excavation, and the archaeological work at the early stages of the exhumation must be careful to preserve the remains in the condition in which they were interred.

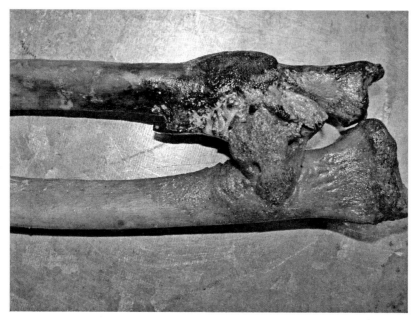

Figure 5-2. Bony mass between radius and ulna from Kosovo indicating previous fracture which was inadequately treated.

Identification, therefore, relies on the careful collection of post-mortem data and its comparison with suitably collected antemortem information. Even in the situation where human rights abuses are being investigated and when many hundreds or even thousands of victims may have been murdered, it behoves all the investigators to do whatever is possible to complete effective identification. This identification may be necessary for the successful prosecution of indicted persons (or even the vindication of the unjustly accused) or it may be part of the closure process for the survivors of atrocities. The need to complete this identification process to the highest standard should not be underestimated and should not be taken for granted. Modern forensic technology allows all but the most deteriorated remains to be identified but this may require the application of extensive resources, both at the time of excavation (through effective archaeological investigation and anthropological examination) as well as later through expensive DNA technology or computing facilities. Human rights abuses may be inflicted upon single individuals, such as in those situations where political internees are abused or killed so that even the single grave may need to be investigated with all the technology available to allow the full forensic pathological investigation of the death to be completed. This will inevitably include the establishment of identity to a level that will withstand rigorous examination by independent forensic reviewers.

The Time or Date of Death

The determination of the postmortem interval is a very important task that must be undertaken early in the forensic investigation of death. It is obvious that by establishing when death occurred at least as accurately as circumstances and the condition of the remains permit, investigators can focus on more relevant issues than would otherwise be the case if the postmortem interval were unknown. There are a number of postmortem changes which are well described and the condition of the body or bodies at exhumation may allow the pathologist or taphonomist (the latter examines environmental effects upon the remains causing changes after death) to estimate when death may have occurred. Early changes such as hypostasis and rigor mortis are unlikely to be present or discernible once the body has been buried and so will rarely be useful observations in the disinterred corpse. Additionally, the cooling of the body is only of practical value in the first 24 hours after death. So it would be very unusual that the time of death could be determined from the physical condition of a body that has been buried after death.

Decomposition, however, is a complex process that includes internal biochemical and cellular breakdown as well as external processes such as intestinal bacteria and fungi and including insect activity (predominantly the effect of maggots) and animal predation. The time scale for decomposition may vary according to changes in soil and environmental conditions as well as varied local factors such as the presence of clothing, the immediate milieu (whether moist or dry) and method of interment. Even in one corpse there may be differing degrees of breakdown between the head and arms which are exposed and the torso and legs which may be protected by clothing. It is imperative for the archaeologist responsible for unearthing remains to remember that the environment in which a body is interred is just as important to the investigating pathologist as it is to the archaeological study. Most bodies will undergo putrefaction, especially if there has not been any attempt at embalming (unlikely in victims of human rights abuses). This process involves a gradual liquefaction of the tissues with production of gas and ultimate loss of soft tissue. In this way, the body may be reduced entirely to skeletal remains. The time taken for this process to finalise depends on many environmental factors. In the buried body, especially important are the temperature, the moisture and the acidity of the soil. When each of these is elevated, putrefaction is enhanced and there may even be demineralisation of bone in particularly acid soils. Therefore, the archaeological examination must include the recording of the burial conditions and this will assist the pathologist in interpreting the state of the remains in respect of the postmortem interval (or at least the post-burial interval). As a corollary, burial in dry conditions, such as sand, may lead to dry decomposition, or mummification. Additionally, in some moist conditions, the fatty tissue may get converted to the waxy substance known as adipocere (Forbes et al., 2005). The rate of decay of bodies buried in earth is much slower than of those in either air or water. Additionally, bodies buried in deep graves tend to remain fairly well-preserved for longer periods than those in shallow graves (such as concealed single homicides). The ground tends to stay colder; it is relatively anaerobic and is not usually affected by rain so stays drier. Therefore knowledge of the burial conditions assists the pathologist in interpreting the physical appearance of the corpse(s) with respect to estimating the postmortem interval.

Animal predation is a natural phenomenon. It may be predation by warm-blooded animals such as rodents or carnivores or it may be the phenomenon of postmortem infestation by insects and arachnids. Archaeological examination must be mindful of the likely involvement of animal predation. The remains that are interred close to the surface of the ground may be unearthed by foraging animals and these may then scatter the bones over an area that corresponds to their normal roaming domain. As well as scattering the bones, the animals may damage them by gnawing and biting. While this is often at the fleshy ends of long bones there may be unusual marks created in flat bones such as the skull. This may confuse the pathologist who is trying to interpret injury patterns and who may regard the linear marks on the bone surface as evidence of sharp force injury such as a knife or bayonet mark. The archaeologist must therefore ensure that the pathologist examining the exhumed remains is made aware of any evidence that suggests the involvement of foraging animals so that any postmortem injuries so caused are not misinterpreted.

Forensic entomology is now a well-established science and any exhumation of previously interred remains must include the study of entomological evidence retrieved from the unearthed body (Byrd and Castner, 2001). The use of the life cycle of infesting insects in calculating postmortem interval is widely accepted but it must be remembered that published insect life cycles do not necessarily apply to all insects in all areas. Before using observations on eggs, maggots, pupae and adults of species in one particular area it is important to remember that insects vary considerably in their distribution and behaviour all over the world and even in smaller areas of one region. Thus, the archaeological excavation must utilise local knowledge of postmortem insect activity before using those observations to calculate postmortem intervals in examined remains. Notwithstanding those limitations, entomological examination, including maggots, live adult insects, spiders, beetles and even pupal cases can assist the pathologist in estimating the postmortem interval and may perhaps aid in the determination whether remains have been buried soon after death or whether they have been buried, exhumed and subsequently reburied elsewhere. As some insects preferentially invade decomposed corpses, their presence may identify a reburial of an already decomposed body. This may have relevance if there is a suspicion that the body of a victim from an execution has been moved from its original site of internment. This has particular relevance to routine police work but may be of value in the special investigations that may follow small numbers of executions. To the practising forensic pathologist, the main limiting factor in this context is the careful collection, preservation and dispatch of suitable samples to an experienced and informed forensic entomologist.

Place of Death

One of the questions often asked of an investigating forensic pathologist is whether the place of body recovery is also the place of death. Clearly if they are the same, then much evidence can be obtained about the crime and about potential offenders by examining the physical evidence located at the site of body retrieval. Even in cases involving the abuse of human rights where mass burial or hurried interment is common there may be useful items of physical evidence that may assist investigators in locating and subsequently convicting perpetrators. The detection of material evidence such as documents, ballistic evidence and other artefacts is usually the province of crime scene examiners of the police or some similar organisation. However, occasionally the pathologist's examination of the remains may uncover physical evidence that facilitates tracking of offenders. Whether victims have been killed at the site of burial may allow subsequent legal investigations to tie the crimes to particular individuals or groups (such as may have been in a particular area at a particular time). So, uncovering physical evidence that confirms the site of killing can assist the pathologist to provide investigators with the reconstruction of the killing time that forms the basis of his investigation. The archaeologist, by examining the method of burial and by carefully locating any evidence that may remain within the gravesite, will help in this process. For example, the description of burial patterns may provide essential evidence of initial events as well as possible excavation and reburials, as was demonstrated during the Balkan wars of the 1990s (Haglund et al., 2001; Dupras et al., 2006). That the bodies may have been buried, exhumed and reburied may be very useful information to the pathologist who is trying to explain to an international tribunal how particular injury patterns observed at autopsy may correlate with alleged events. Once again the involvement of the pathologist at the exhumation and the assistance of the archaeologist at the autopsy will, through the joint approach, allow for a better understanding of the events culminating in a massacre.

The Cause of Death

It is evident that the most important role for the pathologist is to determine the cause of death of the victim(s). Notwithstanding the involvement of the pathologist in other aspects of the investigation as outlined above, the autopsy is regarded as the central pillar of the pathologist's work. The autopsy is properly conducted in a purpose-built mortuary but often in situations where the abuse of human rights is to be investigated (often in or near zones of conflict) facilities are less than perfect. Examples are illustrated in Figures 5-3 and 5-4. Safety and occupational health issues should not be disregarded and are discussed below.

It is clearly beyond the scope of this chapter to discuss the autopsy in detail but it is perhaps worthwhile mentioning some aspects of autopsy practice that are relevant to those situations where human rights abuses are being investigated. Some of these involve the examination of victims of torture or death in custody but these are only relevant to the current volume when death has occurred and burial has preceded the archaeologically controlled exhumation. The first step in the autopsy process is to transport the remains from the site of exhumation to the

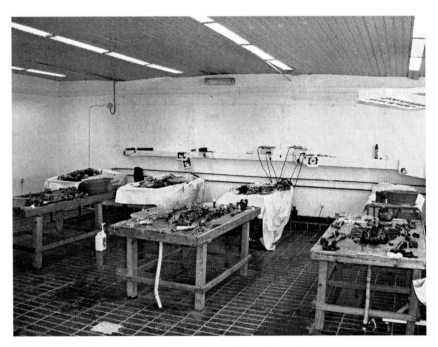

Figure 5-3. The mortuary at Orahovac, Kosovo.

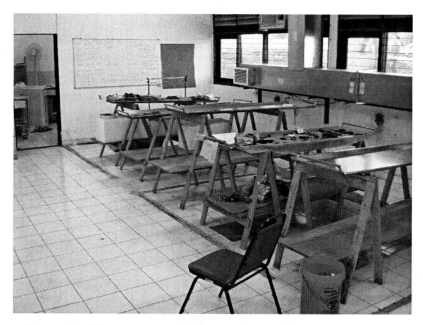

Figure 5-4. The mortuary at the Serious Crimes Unit, Dili, East Timor.

mortuary. This must be conducted under strictly controlled conditions to ensure that the remains are properly collected, collated, bagged and labelled and thereby delivered to the autopsy facility in a manner that prevents any mix-up of specimens. Skeletal remains look remarkably alike so it is essential to ensure proper labelling (Howard et al., 1988). Once the remains are in the possession of the pathologist, he has total control of all subsequent examination.

The remains should be logged in the facility's record system and then photographed. Each set of remains is then assembled with the assistance of a forensic anthropologist should they be fragmented or, more likely, skeletonised. It is prudent to x-ray the remains at an early stage of their examination. This will allow the detection of hazards such as sharp objects, unexploded shells, and bullets or even hand grenades as well as the illustration of projectiles and bony injury that may be important evidence of the crimes being investigated. The remains are probably going to be dirty, having been interred in soils of various types. It will be necessary to clean the bones and this can often be done with simple soap and water, although this depends on available facilities (Fig. 5-5). After the skeletal remains have been cleaned and assembled, there may be the opportunity to conduct a dental examination. This is relevant if

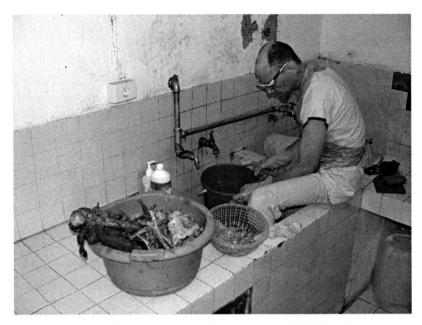

Figure 5-5. Cleaning bones in the mortuary at Dili, East Timor.

identification is to be attempted and if suitable antemortem records are available. The joint examination of the skeletal remains by the anthropologist and the pathologist will allow the maximum interpretation of skeletal damage and the correlation of such injury with other forensic evidence (see Chapter 6 of this volume). For example, if cut marks are identified on bones such as ribs or neck vertebrae then this supports the contention that sharp force injury may have been used such as a machete or bayonet. Likewise the common observation of gunshot wounds of varying sizes, shapes and configurations permits the pathologist to opine as to the firearm used, likely angle and occasionally even distance. Clearly an injury caused by a low velocity handgun which still results in the shattering of a skull or even in an exit wound (such as in an execution) would probably have been inflicted at close range. If a similar weapon only creates an entry wound with little fracturing, no exit wound and a residual projectile, then it is likely to have been used at a greater distance. This has important implications in any legal proceedings that may eventuate following these examinations. So while soft tissue and internal organs are often missing from archaeological specimens, much information can be obtained by professional examination of bony remains. It therefore means that such examinations should be conducted by pathologists with experience in this kind of work. The paucity of skin and lack of soft tissues are conditions with which some forensic pathologists are unfamiliar and recognition of the need for anthropological assistance and archaeological advice is a necessary prerequisite for successful autopsies in these types of cases.

The Manner or Mode of Death

It is part of the pathologist's routine to formulate an opinion about the manner or mode of death. That is, he will indicate whether the findings at autopsy together with any other information that is at hand can allow him to offer an opinion as to whether the death has been as a result of a natural event, an accident, suicide or whether a homicide has been committed. Clearly, in those cases in which forensic archaeology is utilised and especially where the abuse of human rights is an issue, the vast majority of deaths are homicidal. So it is not necessary to further discuss this aspect of the pathologist's role.

Disease and Injury Pattern

Further to the above discussion on the pathologist's role in determining the cause of death, it is usual to complete the examination by investigating and describing all the diseases and injuries that can be observed in the remains. While these may not necessarily contribute directly to death, they may be of assistance in the investigation or may aid in subsequent studies and legal proceedings. For example, investigation of victims of a massacre near the town of Rakos in northwest Kosovo during the war of 1999 revealed that a number of victims had suffered significant peripheral wounds in addition to the usual execution style gunshot wounds in the skull. There had been a claim by the prevailing authorities at the time that many of these individuals had been in a prison which had been bombed by NATO (North Atlantic Treaty Organization) and that the deaths resulted from the bombing. Autopsy demonstration of injuries that would have been incapacitating but not necessarily lethal assisted in refuting the claim and in suggesting that the deaths were in fact executions which followed a variety of other injuries that were most unlikely to be due to the effects of aerial bombing. As such an examination requires skeletal remains that are in a condition that allows this careful study, the excavation of the remains from the burial site must be conducted with great care and with the close cooperation of pathological, archaeological and anthropological investigators.

OCCUPATIONAL HEALTH AND SAFETY

Forensic pathology is a science conducted in conditions and under circumstances that can expose its practitioners to various categories of occupational hazard. Pathologists are very mindful of microbiological dangers that await the unprepared prosector and most modern mortuaries are provided with various levels of protection against potential dangers. Personal protective equipment, designed specially to cater for protection against infection, as well as specific mortuary protocols all serve to allow the pathologist to complete his work with confidence that all reasonable precautions have been undertaken. However, when the pathologist ventures into the world of forensic archaeology, these assumptions must not allow careful safety practises to be forgotten.

Forensic archaeology is about unearthing human remains. Unlike in other branches of archaeology, the biological material may have been interred quite recently. The expectation that the body or bodies will definitely be fully skeletonised, as in the usual archaeological project, must be set aside. The use of archaeological techniques in forensic investigation may result in fully or partially fleshed bodies being examined. So the excavating team should regard the remains as potentially infectious and should make appropriate preparations and take suitable precautions (Skinner, 1987). The simple protocol of wearing gloves and protecting the face will usually suffice. However, it is normal practise to don overalls which either replace or protect normal clothing and which are usually disposable. If the excavation is being conducted in tropical conditions then facilities capable of allowing for excessive heat and humidity should be provided. As these investigations are often conducted in conflict zones this may not always be possible but it is important for the chief investigator to ensure that the welfare of all the team is a top priority (see Chapters 3 and 11 of this volume).

COOPERATION WITH THE SENIOR INVESTIGATOR

The preceding paragraphs serve to highlight perhaps the most important message of this interaction. Where human rights abuses are being investigated, there are often multiple occupant burial sites to be examined. This examination is not the sole province of the investigator, the archaeologist, the anthropologist, the odontologist, the crime scene examiner or the pathologist. The investigation must be a team effort and it is essential that at the early planning stage this cooperative principle is accepted and adopted (Skinner and Sternberg, 2005). There should be a senior investigator whose responsibility is to coordinate the teams and to allocate their different roles and their interaction with other team members and units (for further information see Chapter 4 of this volume). In that way all the participants in the investigation can be assured that their individual roles will be respected and supported and that any information about the burial that is pertinent to the interment and thereby the criminal investigation is not lost in the bureaucratic paper trail that tends to accompany mass investigations.

REFERENCES

Byrd, J.H., and Castner, J.L. (2001). *Forensic entomology: The utility of arthropods in legal investigations.* Boca Raton: CRC Press.

Dupras, T., Schultz, J., Wheeler, S., and Williams, L. (2006). *Forensic recovery of human remains: Archaeological approaches.* Boca Raton: Taylor & Francis.

Forbes, S.L., Stuart, B.H., and Dent, B.B. (2005). The effect of the burial environment on adipocere formation. *Forensic Sci Int, 154*(1):24–34.

Haglund, W.D., Connor, M., and Scott, D.D. (2001). The archaeology of contemporary mass graves. *Historical Archaeology, 35*(1):57–69.

Howard, J.D., Reay, D.T., Haglund, W.D., and Fligner, C.L. (1988). Processing of skeletal remains: A medical examiner's perspective. *Am J Forensic Med Pathol, 9*(3):258–64.

Rudin, N., and Inman, K. (2002). *An introduction to forensic DNA analysis.* 2nd ed. Boca Raton: CRC Press.

Skinner, M. (1987). Planning the archaeological recovery of evidence from recent mass graves. *Forensic Sci Int, 34*(4):267–87.

Skinner, M., and Sterenberg, J. (2005). Turf wars: Authority and responsibility for the investigation of mass graves. *Forensic Sci Int, 151*(2-3):221–32.

Chapter 6

FORENSIC ANTHROPOLOGICAL INTERVENTIONS: CHALLENGES IN THE FIELD AND AT MORTUARY

ROXANA FERLLINI

INTRODUCTION

Within the historical context, the active involvement of forensic anthropologists in human rights investigations commenced in 1984, when the analysis and identification of victims of such abuses was required and applied in a methodical manner in Argentina within investigations pertaining to those who had disappeared during the Dirty War (*Guerra Sucia*) of the late 1970s and early 1980s (for further discussion on this subject see Chapters 1 and 9 of this volume). Since then, the field has grown on a constant basis, proof of this being the increased participation evident in human rights missions conducted by the various non-governmental organizations (NGOs) that have sprung up during the past 22 years, with these NGOs normally working in conjunction with inter-governmental organizations (IGOs). Resultantly, a vast amount of work has been accomplished by forensic anthropologists within such investigations, resulting in the advancement of techniques applied to human identification, and also to approaches by which work is conducted within the mortuary. Methods of coordination, team organization, and importantly, strategies of dealing with local governmental officials and civilian organizations are however, in most instances, dependent on the political climate at the time and the willingness of those involved to cooperate (for actual situations see Chapters 7 and 8 of this volume).

122

The presence of the forensic anthropologist as part of a multidisciplinary forensic team while investigating human rights abuses is of paramount importance, with her or his active participation required not only at the mortuary, but also in the field. With reference to the latter scenario, although as a general rule the forensic anthropologist is most identified with work aimed at the identification of human remains, and in assisting with trauma assessment conducted within the mortuary, their active participation and expertise with the retrieval of human remains may be required and desirable in many cases.

With reference to mortuary work, it is likely that the forensic anthropologist will participate within any given investigation of civilian deaths, and their specific function will be clearly focused upon the most effective manner by which they can assist in fulfilling the objectives deemed to be most important for each particular mission. That is, in some instances, human identification may not be the primary focus of their involvement, but instead, the emphasis may be aiding in the determination of the cause and manner of death. An example of wider involvement could include ascertaining the number of individuals recovered from a mass grave that appeared to have been executed, in order to verify to a tribunal that atrocities had indeed been committed (Sprogøe-Jakobsen et al., 2001).

This chapter will provide an insight into what the forensic anthropologist contributes to international investigations, thus illustrating how their skills provide an important contribution to the investigative process. In particular, their participation in the field and in the mortuary will be highlighted, with an emphasis placed on the particular challenges posed while compiling biological profiles pertaining to individuals from different genetic populations and regions.

INTERVENTION IN THE FIELD AND AT MORTUARY

The active role of the forensic anthropologist varies within different human rights investigations, depending upon the needs that may arise at any given moment, as well as to the specific aspect of job performance that is expected of her or him (for a more detailed description of the various work performed by forensic anthropologists, see Steadman and Haglund, 2005). Because such types of investigations are often completed under demanding budget and time constraints, and at times intense political pressure, it may be necessary for forensic anthropologists to rotate the various tasks that they perform in order to ensure the efficient management of the investigation at hand. Many of these tasks may not be related at all to forensic anthropology, being more in line with administrative functions or different types of hands-on work in the field. Regardless of the manner of work that must be conducted, forensic anthropologists and all other personnel involved in an investigation should be current with all required vaccinations (refer to Chapter 3 of this volume for more detail), which will vary of course, depending upon the part of the world in which their tasks are being conducted.

Participation in the Field

When working within large scale investigations, the search, location, interpretation of the site, and the subsequent recording of human remains in the field should be undertaken by competent forensic archaeologists possessing a solid background in field archaeology that qualifies them to perform such immense and important tasks. Yet, in the case of particular individuals who have ample training in both fields (forensic anthropology and archaeology), such candidates may actively participate in both areas of work.

While working in the field, forensic anthropologists put into practice their knowledge of field archaeology, in addition to their specialized knowledge of bone osteology. For example, in the case of mass graves that contain skeletonized and commingled remains, the exhumation process frequently becomes complicated when attempting to accurately identify the number of individuals present within a given area. The removal of such remains, whilst actively attempting to avoid further commingling, frequently develops into a very demanding task (Ferllini, 1999). If the process is not accomplished properly (as may be the case when anthropologists are asked to participate only in mortuary work by the authorities in the region), such remains will arrive at the mortuary mixed within body bags (Fig. 6-1), which in turn makes the identification process more problematical, the determination of minimum number of individuals (MNI) very challenging, and in some cases, the resulting efforts may not succeed in arriving at appropriate identifications (Fig. 6-2).

Additionally, forensic anthropologists also participate in the recovery of skeletonized human remains that are scattered upon the surface.

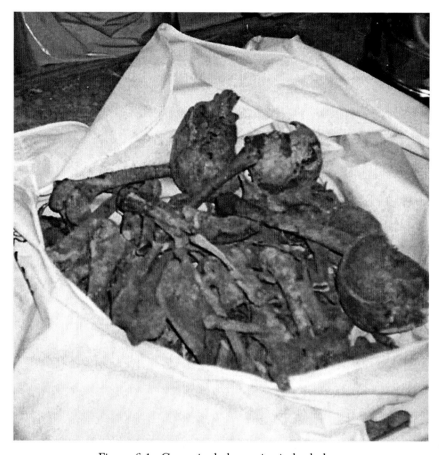

Figure 6-1. Commingled remains in body bag.

In such scenarios, human remains that have been exposed to a variety of taphonomic factors, depending on the geographical location of the site, may have their condition affected in a multitude of ways. If enough time has elapsed for the remains to be skeletonized, disarticulated, and dispersed, may that be the result of animal activity, human intervention, or other factors such as inclined terrains and heavy precipitation, a great amount of effort may be required to affect the location and retrieval of the remains in question. Additionally, the necessity of determining the MNI and whether the remains are actually human in nature is also of importance. It is at this juncture where the careful identification and removal of the skeletonized remains is of great benefit for proper transport to the mortuary for their subsequent processing. Simply being able to effectively differentiate human bones from those of animals may save valuable time, effort and resources later on.

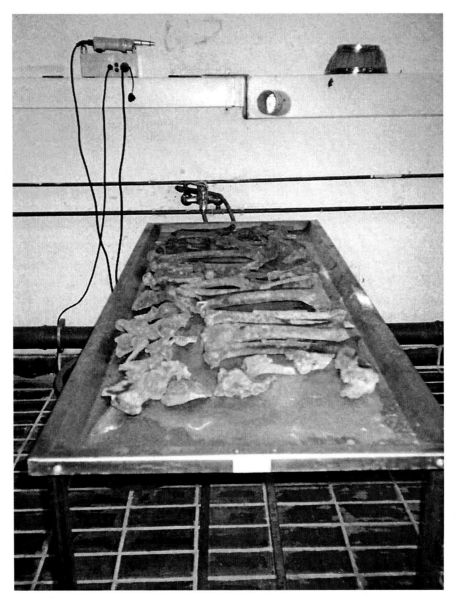

Figure 6-2. Skeletonized remains on mortuary table before determining the MNI.

The above is not intended to imply that anthropologists only work with skeletonized remains. In the field, the condition of bodies being recovered may vary depending on a variety of factors, and forensic anthropologists must be prepared to work with remains that exhibit various degrees of preservation or deterioration. When dealing with a situation where the time lapse between the killing(s) and that of the mission comprises a relatively short time frame, and additionally compounded with climatic conditions that benefit body preservation, such as occurs in the Balkans, it is possible for remains to exhibit a considerable quantity of soft tissue. Saponification (when the fat tissue in the body is converted to adipocere, a whitish waxy substance, after exposure to moisture) may be enhanced with reference to bodies discovered in more humid environments, such as those at the centre of a mass grave, where a micro-environment is created by the humidity of the surrounding body fluids, and by the remains being shielded from external taphonomic factors that would usually contribute to the process of decomposition (Haglund, 2002).

Depending upon the quantity of human remains that are expected to be searched for and retrieved, this factor will serve to determine the number of forensic anthropologists involved at any given time, and will also influence the division of labor as to their participation, both in the field and within the mortuary. With reference to cases in which the work at hand is expected to be extensive, and as is often the case, with restricted time frames, several forensic anthropologists might be present at any given time, with individuals being split into tasks pertaining specifically to fieldwork, or alternatively, duties within the mortuary. On the other hand, in cases where bodies are confirmed to be located in single graves, and when the mission is extended to a more manageable time frame, there may be a requirement for only two forensic anthropologists to be available. What is important, regardless of the circumstances and structure of the mission, is that the work accomplished in the field must ideally be conducted with as appropriate an amount of time as possible, while also ensuring that the remains are retrieved in a proper and thorough manner. This may not always be possible, due to factors such as political circumstances (Simmons, 2007), thereby creating the requirement of performing rescue archaeology, or a general survey, whilst still striving to maintain a minimum core of standards.

Once the remains and other associated items have been recovered, a chain of custody must follow, in which everything at hand should be properly catalogued, stored, and subsequently accessed only by authorized personnel.

Regardless as to where the bodies may be located, care should always be taken with regard to unexploded ordnance. This stark reality of human rights work in the field dictates that under no circumstances should any

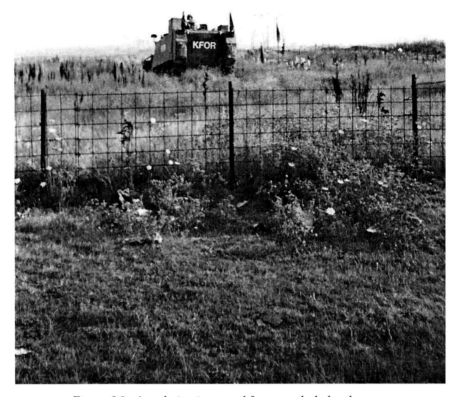

Figure 6-3. Area being inspected for unexploded ordnance.

type of search and rescue be attempted unless the area in question has been properly assessed by qualified personnel, and clear instructions have been conveyed as to when and where it is safe to proceed (Fig. 6-3).

Mortuary Work

The work carried out at the mortuary by forensic anthropologists is most often aimed at conducting a skeletal analysis of the remains, in order to arrive at the required biological profile (sex, age, stature, and any distinctive or individualizing features), and to assess any trauma that might be present, including perimortem trauma, which can aid with the determination of the cause and manner of death. Such work is accomplished in conjunction with the participation of the pathologist, as no postmortem is carried out without the intervention of the latter. The determination of the victims' biological affinity (ancestry) is not usually necessary in such circumstances, since the targeted population is usually known, but there are sometimes exceptions to this rule, as presented within Chapter 5 of this volume.

The settings in which postmortem examinations are conducted vary widely depending on individual circumstances which may involve situations in which the location to be investigated lies far from any type of routine or adequate infrastructure, necessitating the use of portable or prefabricated mortuaries. In other instances, priorities are dictated directly by what might be available in areas that have been affected by conflict; resultantly, this often leads to work being performed in pre-existing autopsy rooms. In such cases, forensic specialists must work as effectively as possible with what might be at hand, be adaptive and innovative, and also improve the installations if and when possible, such as setting up adequate x-ray facilities (Fig. 6-4). Another crucial problem that may be encountered is the lack of a reliable supply of electricity. Power outages can be a commonplace occurrence in some countries, with these events often occurring several times daily. This may serve to create difficulties with work being conducted, by hindering the use of electric equipment in the mortuary, and also the use of computers required to input data that has been compiled throughout the day. A backlog of work may often result, which as a consequence, may accumulate for the following day, or it may imply a longer working day for those who may already be carrying heavy workloads, and who may often be functioning under difficult circumstances. Such an element, in conjunction with often poor internet network services, also serves to hamper the communication process with other professionals and organizations residing outside of the area in question, but whom may also be directly involved in the investigative process.

In particularly difficult circumstances, work may have to actually be accomplished whilst in the field, due to the location of the site being investigated; that is, working without any adequate facilities nearby, with the only possibility being the establishment of a portable mortuary, containing only a very basic infrastructure. This creates the requirement of setting up the mortuary from scratch, and some of the anthropologists involved in the mission will be required to assess what materials are most necessary for their day-to-day work. Such circumstances are not easy because all of those involved must use their ingenuity in order to accomplish the task at hand, without compromising the quality of their work and the eventual results. An excellent example of this would be work conducted in Kibuye, Rwanda, when existing building structures were converted

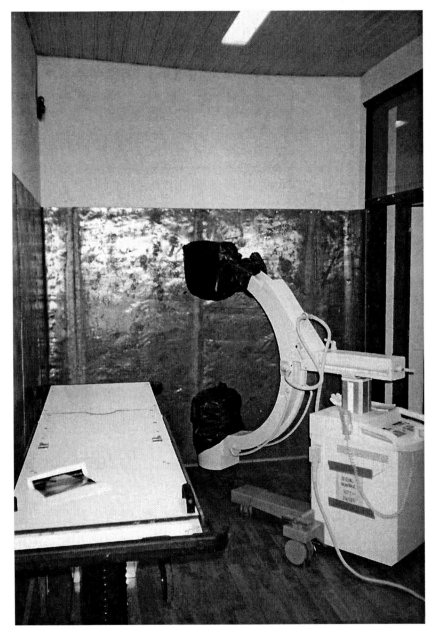

Figure 6-4. Kosovo: x-ray room set up within a pre-existing autopsy area.

into office spaces, and an inflatable mortuary was erected. The necessary efforts were completed with a minimum of equipment, and yet the
desired quality of the work was fully attained (Ferllini, 1999; Koff, 2004).

Another approach is the utilization of a mobile autopsy, in situations when the infrastructure is minimal and the necessary work must be performed in the open air; such a manner of arrangement was utilized by the Danish-Swedish forensic teams in Kosovo. According to Sprogøe-Jakobsen et al. (2001), mobile teams have the advantage of moving efficiently from one area to another throughout a vast region, working on relatively small sites in which small quantities of single graves require exhumation, and where the determination of the cause and manner of death is the main aim of the forensic examinations. Although identification may not in these circumstances be the focal point, in the case of the Danish-Swedish team, one anthropologist was always present during postmortem examinations.

With regard to the required infrastructure for the forensic anthropologist, this would normally include an area with appropriate supplies to conduct maceration if necessary (running water, pans, a stove, plastic containers, scalpels, tweezers among other items, although some techniques are not recommended when DNA sampling is required – see DNA analysis section in this chapter), reference materials, x-ray facilities, calipers (spreading and sliding), an osteometric board, and concise but efficient postmortem protocols. Such a list would of course vary depending upon the circumstances involved.

The protocols to be utilized, which may often be created by one or a few individuals, can serve to create confusion at times, due to the differences in the academic backgrounds of each anthropologist. That is, whilst in the Americas, the academic formation tends to be similar throughout, with a major influence coming from North America. In other regions, such as Europe, the educational background varies widely, and hence the approaches taken at the mortuary will also vary (Brickley and Ferllini, 2007; Skinner et al., 2003). As a consequence during international missions, because the teams are often composed of individuals from a variety of different countries, and hence many backgrounds, the additional barrier of language may also create difficulties with respect to basic communication, and to the set standards to be agreed upon (author's personal observation).

Not only are working conditions a concern for those involved, but storage is also an important issue that needs to be given due consideration. When the remains being recovered are in a state of decomposition, ideally they should be stored in refrigerated conditions (Fig. 6-5). However, in many situations this may not be possible, and storage may

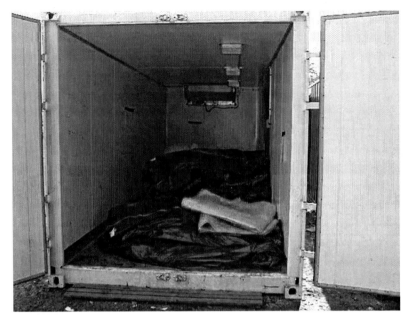

Figure 6-5. Refrigerated storage container with individual body bags.

need to be accomplished in empty buildings that are accessible, and in which the process of decomposition will of course continue.

It is clear that work in such unusual circumstances, due to the nature of human rights missions, can often create some stresses on those conducting the necessary tasks. A number of negative aspects are encountered in mortuary work, one in particular being the proximity of grieving relatives and friends in some instances, which can make work difficult to perform, and can also be a source of distraction, mostly due to the emotional tension and outbursts expected in such situations. Additionally, the uneasiness that results from badly decomposed bodies being observed by such distraught individuals, as may often occur at times whilst in the field, is another factor to consider (Sprogøe-Jakobsen et al., 2001; author's personal observation).

IDENTIFICATION AND POPULATION SPECIFICS

Challenges in Biological Profiling

In order for the forensic anthropologist to achieve the identification of human remains, a biological profile must be conducted on each victim through osteological analysis. To obtain such a profile, a given methodology is required. However, such terms of reference must be proven to have been adequately researched and also published after a careful peer review. Such methods will in time become accepted as standards, and will be routinely applied in forensic cases. Nonetheless, even though such applications may become widely accepted, it needs to be emphasized that their accuracy when applied can only be attained with reference to individuals who share the same genetic derivation as the population utilized to conduct the research and development of the methods being employed. Hence, the identification process can be achieved with accuracy only when working with populations that have been properly studied, and their developmental and morphological variability known. However, on the other hand, it can be a demanding process for any forensic anthropologist when having to examine remains from population groups that have not been previously studied, or that the anthropologist may not have previous experience with. Consequently, the profiling process is not without its problems when working with remains of which the range of variability is not known, creating the potential for skewed and inaccurate results. As stated by Djuric (2004), without local identification standards, the results obtained from a biological profile may be biased. Thus, it is important that such standards be actively developed in order to achieve results of high quality.

It frequently transpires in the field of human rights investigations that the victims that require identification are more often than not representative of populations that have never been formally studied and researched for skeletal variations, growth patterns and morphological characteristics. This is not to suggest that work done in the past under such circumstances is not valid, or to imply that the results so far achieved must be incorrect; as a general rule, the standards applied in a broad sense do tend to encompass those found in the remains of different genetic make-ups. Yet, the use of population specific methods are best desired, and recently, research has been conducted in order to achieve specific standards for different populations (Schaefer and Black, 2005).

In order to address this problem with populations that have been victims of human rights abuses, research in recent years has been aimed at developing methods appropriate to some of these groups. Such research must be compiled from contemporary forensic origins, in order to have a valid application (Frutos, 2002). In this respect, the author wishes to note and emphasize that such studies should be conducted at all times under strict and appropriate ethical codes and guidelines, with the full approval of family members, and for the analysis to be conducted with solely scientific aims.

Additionally, there are two problems which may place limitations upon the identification process; the first is encountered when identifying a group of individuals coming from a single context find, and who share several biological characteristics amongst them, such an identical sex ratio, and being of similar age and stature. Such a type of circumstance has been encountered in the Balkan region (Komar, 2003) where the victims have often been statistically similar males, often from extended families, and hence sharing similar characteristics. The second problem pertains to the availability of antemortem data, obtained either through interviews with relatives and friends of the deceased, or through formal medical or dental records, such as radiographs (Angyal and Derczy, 1998; Thompson and Puxley, 2006) and DNA analysis. In the first instance, this is referred to as presumptive identification (Simmons and Haglund, 2005) in which a physical description of the individual, information on health-related issues, and also data pertaining to clothing worn the last time the victim was seen alive can be obtained. In the latter case, this is referred to as positive identification, but records of this nature are not routinely used, as few records of any nature are kept in many of the regions where such types of investigations take place (Primorac et al., 1996).

A word of caution should be made, however, on the use of clothing as part of the identification process. This can be a limiting factor in certain circumstances, such as after the Rwandan genocide of 1994. Due to the low number of survivors, such an exercise proved to be of limited success (Koff, 2004; Ferllini, 1999). Nonetheless, such an approach may often produce positive results if survivors are available for interviews. Matches of verbal description of the individuals in question with the biological profiles obtained may then be possible in some cases (see Fig. 6-6).

Sex Determination

Sex determination of bodies that are highly decomposed must be conducted based on skeletal analysis, either through morphological assessment or through metric data. Either method will reflect the sexual dimorphism present in any given population, that is, the different characteristics between male and female in size and proportions. These differences are not shared by all populations, and when improperly used,

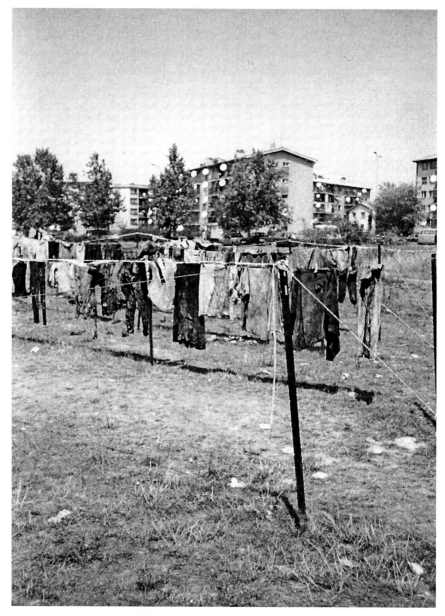

Figure 6-6. Clothing which has been removed from the bodies, cleaned and left to dry for future identification by family members.

the results may be skewed; hence their utilization must be used with caution. Problems may arise in that depending on the sex of the individual, the determination of age and stature will be accomplished by using the appropriate methods designed for males and females respectively (Slaus et al., 2003). As such, forensic anthropologists should be aware when possible of specific variants between males and females for the population with which they are working, in order to assess a biological profile with proper accuracy, and thereby avoid potential bias. However, many populations have not yet been studied and documented, therefore creating a possible lack of standards that could be applied during the identification process. Yet, an important advantage to any forensic anthropologist when conducting identifications is to have first-hand knowledge of the population at hand. While working in different regions of the world for sufficient periods of time, anthropologists can develop knowledge on the specific morphological characteristics that can help distinguish between the sexes, the developmental rates and the aging process associated with the group being analyzed, a great advantage when the profiling is being accomplished along with established methodologies.

Determination of the sex of an individual can be accomplished with a high degree of confidence based upon the morphological characteristics present in the cranium, mandible and pelvis (Stewart, 1979; Bass, 1995). It should be noted that while the cranium and mandible can be used to determine sex, many of the victims of human rights violations, as observed by the author, may exhibit severe trauma to the head and facial region, which may make an accurate assessment difficult, if not impossible at times.

In the area of metric assessment, research in recent years has produced a series of discriminant functions for various populations, such as those in the Balkans and Guatemala. Slaus et al. (2003) created discriminant functions to be applied to incomplete and complete femora from the Croatian population, with a high percentage rate of success. Attempts at developing such techniques have also been approached by Frutos (2002; 2005) with reference to the Guatemalan rural population, which has suffered from severe human rights abuses during the past three decades. Specifically, sex determination through metrics, using the clavicle and scapula, has been attained for a rural Guatemalan population, providing a high rate of success. When the same specimens were compared with standards provided for North Americans, the rate of success in determining the sex was considerably lower (Frutos, 2002). Frutos (2005) also developed a discriminant function for sex determination utilizing the humerus, demonstrating that bone dimensions may vary widely between populations. The noted differences are produced by factors that influence the development at the inter and intra population level, such as the nutritional condition of an individual during the developmental years, level of activity, and genetic make-up, among other factors (Frutos, 2005). A word of caution, as observed by the author; the implementation of craniometrics and the use of FORDISC® (Owsley and Jantz, 1996) to determine sex may produce negative results when applied to populations that have not been included within the statistical program (L'engle Williams et al., 2005).

Age Estimation

Age estimation is not without its problems due to the specific variability that a population may exhibit, either from genetic and/or environmental factors (geographical setting, nutrition, social status, stress levels, working conditions, among others) which play in the development of the individuals in a specific population, and hence influencing the aging processes. Such variables are numerous, with many not being well understood. Most studies conducted on age estimation have been based on western populations which are not compatible to populations from other areas of the world, creating a high probability of unreliable results when applied to non-western populations (Schmitt, 2004).

However, studies have been conducted in order to better understand specific populations. In the case of population groups from the Balkan region, a study was conducted by Schaefer and Black (2005) on the epiphyseal union of juveniles from Bosnia. These were compared to juveniles from North America, in order to assess their rate of maturation. The results indicate that while standards from the US-based studies can be applied to those from Bosnia, the rate of maturation on the latter was two to three years sooner than their North American counterparts. This study demonstrates that while the American standards can be applied, a more accurate result can be attained if Bosnian specifics are to be utilized.

Age estimation in adults is rather limited in that the developmental processes have ceased at the dental level, and most bone fusion also ceases after the age of 30. One of the methods widely utilized for estimating adult age is the Suchey-Brooks method, based on the morphological changes observed on the pubic symphysis (Katz and Suchey, 1986; Katz and Suchey, 1989; Klepinger et al., 1992; Bass, 1995). While the research conducted to produce this method included individuals from different ancestries and backgrounds, the method is not free of error. This particular method was applied on bodies of known age in Belgrade by Djuric et al. (2003), and by Schmitt (2004) in Thailand, in order to test its reliability within the Balkan and Thai populations. The findings in both studies illustrated that the method is not reliable when applied to other populations not represented within the original re-search sample, and in non-western populations.

While the Balkan population is being studied in order to better un-derstand how age estimation can be more accurately assessed by devel-oping, where possible, specific population standards, other populations have received little or no attention at all in the field of research. An ex-ample of such a situation would be some African populations that reside in areas where human rights abuses have occurred or continue to occur, and yet no studies have been conducted to produce much needed stan-dards that could apply to them. The reasons for this are varied, includ-ing circumstances where such research cannot be conducted due to logistical problems and insecure settings.

The process of age estimation should be accomplished with reference to all available markers, bone and/or teeth, in order to obtain a range for the estimated age on a particular individual, yet as stated by Sim-mons and Haglund (2005) age can be estimated but without the results being precise; this, compounded with a lack of population standards, makes the work of the anthropologist much more challenging.

Determining Stature

The stature of a given population is subject to genetic factors, in ad-dition to many environmental issues already cited in this chapter. At the individual level, the socio-economic strata will have an influence re-garding access to adequate nutrition and medical attention, factors which may serve to influence the growth and height attained during the developmental period. Consequentially, populations throughout the world do exhibit different long bone proportions, and the use of inade-quate stature formulae in a given population may result in either an under or overestimate of the actual height of the body being analyzed.

Initially, studies were conducted in the US, including the early work done by Trotter and Gleser (1952); however, most efforts have been fo-cused on the American white and black population, including research aimed at developing regression formulae for incomplete limb bones

(Steele and Bramblett, 1988; Simmons, et al., 1990; Holland, 1992). As such, caution should be applied in other areas of the world when attempting to ascertain stature from limb bones. Unlike age estimation, stature can be precise if appropriate information is at hand for the population to which the victims belonged (Simmons and Haglund, 2005). Wright and Vázquez (2003) studied the estimation of fragmented long bones from a Guatemalan Mayan population. Their findings pointed to a higher rate of success when the specific population formulae were applied versus those made for a different population. For the Balkan region, Ross and Konigsberg (2002) developed formulae based on Bosnian and Croatian remains, demonstrating that the stature could be underestimated if formulae designed for Western whites were applied.

The verification of stature results has to be based on antemortem information, either from family or friends (Dujiric, 2004), or from formal documents such as passports, driver's licenses or military records. In the former case, the information received may not be reliable, since it is based on memory and often the height is compared against another person or structure (author's observation). The latter is not usually an option, since most would not have such records.

Individualizing Traits

There are many individualizing traits that can be utilized for identification, such as antemortem trauma, where the bone morphology has been altered (Fig. 6-7) and evidence of bone remodelling is present. Bone pathologies, such as diffused idiopathic skeletal hyperostosis (DISH), rheumatoid arthritis and gout, are conditions that can aid in the identification process (Ortner and Putschar, 1981; for more detailed descriptions of the application of ostepathologies within the field of forensics, consult Warren and Falsetti, 1999; Cunha and Pinheiro, 2007; Djuric, 2004; Pinheiro et al., 2004). Additionally, dental traits, and treatment received are often of important value in the identification process. It is here where the input of the investigative personnel can coordinate a database where the information received from interviews and other sources can be compared to information resulting from the mortuary findings. As such, it is hoped that a compatibility with both sets of data is made and identifications can be achieved (Fig. 6-7), or at best, work to create a stronger case before other methods are applied. This is why a daily meeting should be scheduled between individuals of any working

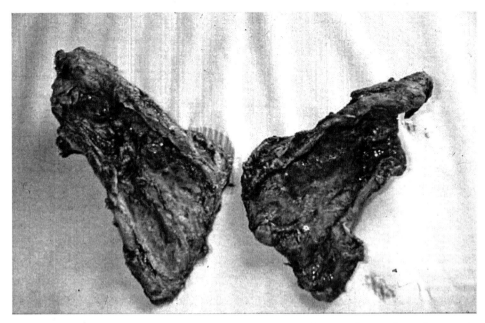

Figure 6-7. Scapulae taken from a civil war victim. Note the atrophy on the right scapula due to antemortem trauma. This particular injury aided in the identification of the victim.

group, in order to inform each other of new data and other developments that may be of consequence.

Unlike medical conditions in which pain and deformities could be easily noted or recalled by memory, specifics on dental work are seldom known by others; in addition, dental identification is extremely limited in these types of circumstances and more often than not, never utilized. In the Balkans, for example, the dental condition in many victims may be extremely poor, and loss of teeth at an early age is not uncommon; when treatments are observed, antemortem data may not be available.

DNA Analysis

Although the application of DNA analysis in the field of human rights investigations has increased considerably, it is not always as successful as is generally perceived. DNA examination, while often serving to positively identify an individual or sort out commingled remains, can often experience limitations, such as those encountered in the Rwandan genocide, where entire families were massacred; or in the case of

Srebrenica, in Bosnia, where many of those killed were from extended families, thereby creating the problem of identifying closely-related individuals, such as the case of siblings; in the latter case, these individuals would be equally related to their biological parents (Koff, 2004; Schaefer and Black, 2005).

DNA analysis, utilizing nuclear and mitochondrial (mtDNA) markers began to be applied in the first part of the 1990s with the aim of obtaining a positive identification (Hagelberg et al., 1991). After soft tissue decomposition, normally bone and teeth are the elements available for DNA testing. Of the two, the teeth are the most reliable in two aspects; firstly, they survive longer than bone; secondly, they provide, as a general rule, a better quality yield of DNA, even in relation to remains that may have been buried for many years (Boles et al., 1995). Techniques have improved over the years, and DNA testing can now be conducted even on degraded material, with a positive rate of success.

A point of caution here; maceration is frequently employed in the autopsy room in order to access the bone to evaluate aspects of the biological profile as well as to aid in examining areas exhibiting trauma. Some of the techniques employed to remove soft tissue may cause damage to the chemical component of bone, which in turn will affect the quality and quantity of the DNA extracted. According to Steadman et al. (2006) the maceration technique that most affects the quantity and quality of nuclear DNA extraction for analysis is that of bleaching; while the results obtained by Arismendi et al. (2004) indicate that prolonged exposure to high temperatures, as in boiling, can have a negative effect on the results obtained from DNA analysis. Hence, as a general practice, the removal of a bone sample (usually from the femur) and also a tooth at the commencement of an autopsy procedure is commonly practiced.

Trauma Assessment

Trauma assessment is a vital part of any postmortem examination in human rights investigations, and the forensic anthropologist can play an important role by working in conjunction with the forensic pathologist. Specifically, the intervention of the forensic anthropologist consists of maceration (if needed), and reconstruction and interpretation, but their work is not necessarily accomplished in these specific steps. In cases where bodies exhibit a degree of decomposing soft tissue or adipocere (Fig. 6-8), tissue removal may be required, and this may be conducted

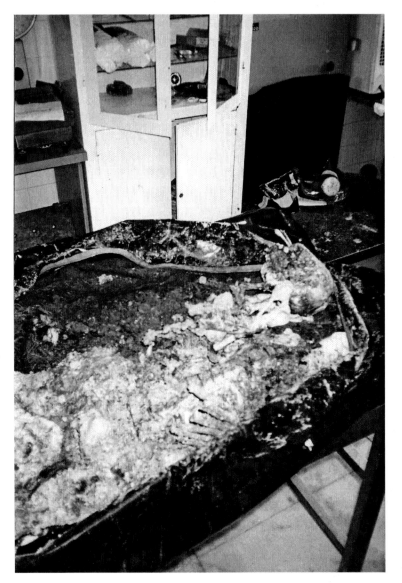

Figure 6-8. Body being prepared for autopsy exhibiting adipocere.

by hand by an experienced anthropologist, who has the expertise to do so without altering the area in question. It is also vitally important that tissue removal should be performed by an individual who is fully competent with the appropriate techniques, and who is aware that any marks left on the bones by the process create a postmortem artifact, thereby altering the context of the trauma being analyzed. If any bones have been shattered due to the trauma, *refitting* of the dislodged segments with appropriate adhesive will be required. Once in place, the interpretation of the trauma can then be more readily ascertained. This process is made possible by understanding bone modification under specific circumstances, that is, a distinction that can be made between trauma that is antemortem, perimortem or postmortem.

Perimortem trauma, which occurs at or around the time of death, is used to determine the cause of death. Under this category, the anthropologist, as a general rule, seeks evidence of three types of trauma; those caused by sharp force, inflicted by objects such as a knife or hatchet producing stabs, cuts or chop actions (Galloway, 1999; DiMaio and DiMaio, 1989). The next category is that of blunt force, caused by heavy objects such as a hammer or rifle butt, which serve to cause radiating fractures and sometimes fragmentation. Finally, gunshot wounds may be evident, a type of trauma frequently encountered in some parts of the world such as the Balkans. Knowledge of ballistics is also desirable in order to interpret the trauma present, the events surrounding the shooting(s) and to be able to recognize associated secondary fractures visible upon the victims (Warren, 2007).

When the area in question has been shattered due to the nature of the trauma, the forensic anthropologist is able to piece the various sections back together, which in some cases involves fragments that may be quite small. This process aids the work of the forensic pathologist, by having the bone reconstructed to its anatomical form, or as close as possible, enabling an accurate determination of the cause of death. It should be made clear that the determination of the cause of death is ascertained by the pathologist and not by the forensic anthropologist. The latter's role, as previously stated, would be to aid with reconstructions if necessary, and also assisting with the interpretation of the injury (or injuries) at hand.

Postmortem trauma often occurs as a result of the improper handling of remains during the exhumation process, and exemplifies the need for qualified and experienced forensic archaeologists and anthropologists to be present during the excavation procedures, thereby ensuring the proper treatment of human remains that may be skeletonized, or in various stages of decomposition. When bone suffers postmortem breakage, one of the manners of determining if such damage is postmortem in nature is to search for sharp jagged edges on the rim of the breakage; this is a result of the brittleness of the bone after the soft tissues have decomposed and the bone has dried out (Fig. 6-9). Additionally, a

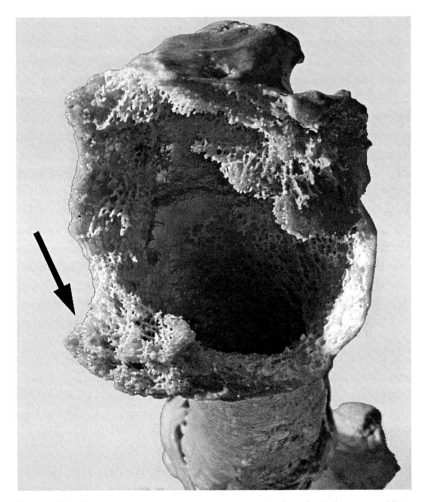

Figure 6-9. Postmortem trauma present at proximal end of a humerus. Note the sharp edges due to bone brittleness after losing its natural moisture (Courtesy of W. Birch, Anatomy Laboratory, University College London).

difference in color along the edges of the affected area will be evident in contrast to the rest of the bone, since the exposure of the bone to soil and other environmental factors will have been different.

DISCUSSION

The above demonstrates the two main roles which the forensic anthropologist serves to provide during human rights missions, and draws attention to the many challenges that can be encountered in the field, and within the mortuary, whilst attempting to obtain an accurate biological profile of the victims. Some of the drawbacks in obtaining a positive identification may be minimized by holding meetings on a regular basis to discuss progress made, goals attained, and any new information obtained from relatives that could be of assistance to the identification process. This type of open information is of value to both the anthropologist and the pathologist, who should always work together during the postmortem, and also to other authorities that are involved in the investigation.

It is hoped that more research will be conducted on population specific methods, especially within areas where no previous studies have been attempted, and where such data is much required.

ACKNOWLEDGMENT

I wish to give special thanks to those who read the various drafts of this chapter, and gave their valuable comments; to Mr. S. Laidlaw, photographer at the Institute of Archaeology, University College London, for his help in preparing the illustrations for this chapter, and to Professor S. Black for her permission to publish the photographs presented here, some taken while working for the Centre for International Forensic Assistance (CIFA). Finally, I wish to thank Dr. M. Brickley of the University of Birmingham for her comments on paleopathologies and their application to human identification.

REFERENCES

Angyal, M., and Derczy, K. (1998). Personal identification on the basis of antemortem and postmortem radiographs. *J. Forensic Sciences, 43*(5):1089–1093.

Arismendi, J., Baker, L., and Matteson, K. (2004). Effects of processing techniques on the forensic DNA analysis of human skeletal remains. *J. Forensic Sciences, 49*(5):930–934.

Bass, W. (1995). *Human osteology. A laboratory and field manual.* Missouri: Archaeological Society Inc.

Boles, T.C., Snow, C., and Stover, E. (1995). Forensic DNA testing on skeletal remains from mass graves: A pilot project in Guatemala. *J. Forensic Sciences 40*(3):349–355.

Brickley, M. and Ferllini, R. (2007). Forensic anthropology: Developments in two continents. In *Forensic anthropology: Case studies from Europe*, Brickley, M., and Ferllini, R. (Eds.). Springfield: Charles C Thomas. In press.

Cunha, E., and Pinheiro, J. (2007). Forensic anthropology in Portugal: Form current practice to future challenges. In *Forensic anthropology: Case studies from Europe*, Brickley, M., and Ferllini, R. (Eds.). Springfield: Charles C Thomas. In press.

DiMaio, D.J., and DiMaio, V.J.M. (1989). *Forensic pathology.* New York: Elsevier.

Djuric, M. (2004). Anthropological data in individualization of skeletal remains from a forensic context in Kosovo. A case history. *J. Forensic Sciences, 49*(3):464–468.

Djuric, M., Djonic, D., Rakocevic, Z., and Nikolic, S. (2003). Evaluation of Suchey-Brooks methods for aging skeletons in the Balkans. *Forensic Science International 136*(Suppl):172.

Ferllini, R. (1999). The role of forensic anthropology in human rights issues. In *Forensic osteological analysis: A book of case studies*, Fairgrieve, C.I. (Ed.). Springfield: Charles C Thomas Publishers, pp. 287–302.

Frutos, L.R. (2002). Determination of sex from the clavicle and scapula in a Guatemalan contemporary rural indigenous population. *American J. Forensic Medicine and Pathology 23*(3):284–288.

Frutos, L.R. (2005). Metric determination of sex from the humerus in a Guatemalan forensic sample. *Forensic Science International, 147*(2-3):153–157.

Galloway, A. (Ed.) (1999). *Broken bones: Anthropological analysis of blunt force trauma.* Springfield: Charles C Thomas.

Hagelberg, E., Gray, I. and Jeffreys, A. (1991). Identification of the skeletal remains of a murder victim by DNA analysis. *Nature 352*(6334):427–429.

Haglund, W. (2002). Recent mass graves: An introduction. In *Advances in forensic taphonomy: Method, theory and archaeological perspectives*, Haglund, W.D., and Sorg, M.H. (Eds.). Boca Raton: CRC Press, pp. 243–261.

Holland, T. (1992). Estimation of adult stature from fragmentary tibias. *J. Forensic Sciences, 37*(5):1223–1229.

Katz, D., and Suchey, J. (1986). Age determination of the male Os Pubis. *American Journal of Physical Anthropology, 69*:427–435.

Katz, D., and Suchey, J. (1989). Race differences in pubic symphyseal aging patterns in the male. *American Journal of Physical Anthropology 80*(2):167–172.

Klepinger, L., Katz, D., Micozzi, M., and Carroll, L. (1992). Evaluation of cast methods for estimating age from the *Os Pubis. J. Forensic Sciences, 37*(3):763–770.

Koff, C. (2004). *The bone woman: Among the dead in Rwanda, Bosnia, Croatia and Kosovo.* London: Atlantic Book.

Komar, D. (2003). Lessons from Srebrenica: The contributions and limitations of physical anthropology in identifying victims of war crime. *J. Forensic Sciences 48*(4):713–716.

L'engle Williams, F., Belcher, R., and Armelagos, G. (2005). Forensic misclassification of ancient Nubian Crania: Implications for assumptions about human variation. *Current Anthropology 46*(2):340–346.

Ortner, D.J., and Putschar, W.G.J. (1981). *Identification of pathological conditions in human skeletal remains.* Washington, D.C.: Smithsonian Institution.

Owsley, S.D., and Jantz, R.L. (1996). *FORDISC 2.0: Personal computer forensic discriminant functions.* Knoxville: University of Tennessee.

Pinheiro, J., Cunha, E., Cordeiro, C., and Vieira, N. (2004). Bridging the gap between forensic anthropology and osteoarchaeology – A case of vascular pathology. *Int. J. Osteoarchaology, 14*:137–144.

Primorac, D., Adelinović, S., Definis-gojanović, M., Drmie, I., Rezie, B., Baden, M., Kennedy, M., Schanfield, M., Skakel, S., and Lee, H. (1996). Identification of war victims from mass graves in Croatia, Bosnia, and Herzegovina by the use of standard forensic methods and DNA typing. *J. Forensic Sciences, 41*(5):891–894.

Ross, A.H., and Konigsberg, L.W. (2002). New formulae for estimating stature in the Balkans. *J. Forensic Sciences, 47*(1):165–167.

Schaefer, M.C., and Black, S.M. (2005). Comparison of ages of epiphyseal union in North American and Bosnian skeletal material. *J. Forensic Sciences, 50*(4):777–783.

Schmitt, A. (2004). Age-at-Death assessment using the *Os Pubis* and the auricular surface of the illium: A test on an identified Asian sample. *Int. J. Osteoarchaeology, 14*:1–6.

Simmons, T. (2007). Fleeing Srebrinica: A surprise attack on a group of men and boys in the moutains. In *Forensic anthropology: Case studies from Europe*, Brickley, M., and Ferllini, R. (Eds.). Springfield: Charles C Thomas. In press.

Simmons, T., and Haglund, W. (2005). Anthropology in a forensic context. In *Forensic archaeology: Advances in theory and practice*, Hunter, J., and Cox, M. (Eds.). London: Routledge, pp. 159–176.

Simmons, T., Jantz, M., and Bass, W. (1990). Stature estimation from fragmentary femora: A revision of the Steele method. *J. Forensic Sciences, 35*(3):628–636.

Skinner, M., Alempijevic, D., and Djuric-Srejic, M. (2003). Guidelines for international forensic bio-archaeology monitors of mass grave exhumations. *Forensic Science International, 134*:81–92.

Slaus, M., Strinović, D., Skavić, J., and Potrevecki, V. (2003). Discriminant function sexing fragmentary and complete femora: Standards for contemporary Croatia. *J. Forensic Sciences, 48*(3):509–512.

Sprogøe-Jakobsen, S., Eriksson, A., Hougen, H.P., Knudsen, P.J., Leth, P., and Lynnerup, N. (2001). Mobile autopsy teams in the investigation of war crimes in Kosovo. *J. Forensic Sciences, 46*(6):1392–1396.

Steadman, D. W., Diantonio, L., Wilson, J., Sheridan, K., and Tammariello, S. (2006). The effects of chemical and heat maceration techniques on the recovery of nuclear and mitochondrial DNA from bone. *J. Forensic Sciences, 51*(1):11–17.

Steadman, D.W., and Haglund, W. (2005). The scope of anthropological contributions to human rights investigations. *J. Forensic Sciences, 50*(1):23–30.

Steele, D.G., and Bramblett, C.A. (1988). *The anatomy and biology of the human skeleton.* College Station: Texas A&M University Press.

Thompson, T.J.U., and Puxley, A. (2006). Personal effects. In *Forensic human identification: An introduction*, Thompson, T.J.U., and Black, S.M. (Eds.). Boca Raton: CRC Press, pp. 365–377.

Warren, M. (2007). Interpreting gunshot wounds in the Balkans: Evidence for genocide. In *Forensic anthropology: Case studies from Europe*, Brickley, M., and Ferllini, R. (Eds.). Springfield: Charles C Thomas. In press.

Warren, M., and Falsetti, A. (1999). Dish, rats, and a rolex. In *Forensic osteological analysis: A book of case studies*, Fairgrieve, S. (Ed.). Springfield: Charles C Thomas, pp. 79–88.

Wright, L.E., and Vázquez, M.A. (2003). Estimating the length of incomplete long bones: Forensic standards from Guatemala. *American Journal of Physical Anthropology 120*(3):233–251.

Chapter 7

FORENSIC ANTHROPOLOGY IN BOSNIA AND HERZEGOVINA: THEORY AND PRACTICE AMIDST POLITICS AND EGOS

Eva-Elvira Klonowski

INTRODUCTION

Mankind has waged war for centuries, but the advent of the twentieth century ushered in an age of genocide, atrocities and barbarism, and resultantly, frequent abuses of human rights and mass graves. It was the century that gestated two horrifying world wars as well as many other wars and bloody conflicts in different countries across the globe. The twentieth century introduced us to and created new words and policies such as genocide, holocaust, gulags, ethnic cleansing or "the disappeared," such terms being invented to express the horror of the deaths of millions of innocent people whose only mistake was to be born in the wrong time and in the wrong place. This global carnival of death left as its legacy millions of names on lists of missing persons. The worst atrocities were committed against Armenians in Turkey, the Jews across Europe, Cambodians, Tutsis in Rwanda, the populations of the former Soviet Union, Argentina, Guatemala, in almost all regions of the former Yugoslavia and in many other countries. What remained afterwards were hidden mass graves, human remains scattered in the fields and within forests, and a living legacy of countless suffering families.

The first recorded opening of mass graves occurred during World War II. In the spring of 1940 as many as 15,000 Polish Army officers and prisoners of war (POWs) were executed by the Soviet KGB forces.

They were buried secretly in mass graves, some located in the Katyn Forest, near the town of Smolensk, in the former Soviet Republic of Belarus. Three years later, this burial site was detected by Germans who, between the 13th of April and the 7th of June 1943, exhumed 4,143 bodies from seven mass graves. Exhumations of the eighth and final grave, consisting of about 260 bodies, were prevented by weather conditions. During the two months of exhumations and examinations, approximately 3,000 remains were identified (Madajczyk, 1989; Paul, 1991).

Since the conclusion of the Second World War in 1945, only the geographic locations of wars have changed. During the past decades, civil wars in Central and South America, Asia, Africa and in the 1990s in Europe, have taken the lives of millions of people.

After the Holocaust, the worst genocide in Europe took place during the war of 1992–1995 within the territory of the former Yugoslavia, in Bosnia and Herzegovina. Under the guise of "ethnic cleansing," over one million people were expelled from their houses and became refugees; while more than a hundred thousand lost their lives (Skirbič, 2006). After the war in Bosnia and Herzegovina concluded, approximately thirty thousand people were unaccounted for. They were buried in mass graves, dumped into caves (Klonowski, 2007), burned in their homes, or left lying on the ground in the forests, fields or hills of their homeland waiting to be discovered, identified, and returned to their families for proper burial.

Beginning in late 1995, the first exhumations in the territory of Bosnia and Herzegovina (BiH) commenced. No one was prepared for the task of exhuming the incomprehensible number of bodies or skeletal remains. During the first year of exhumations, almost 2,000 remains were recovered in BiH, and this was but a fraction of those reported missing. Since then, and until 2006, hundreds of all manners of graves were opened, and thousands of human remains recovered.

The main purpose of opening the mass graves or collecting unburied surface remains was, and still is, to effect positive identifications of the deceased, and to return their remains to grieving families.

HISTORICAL BACKGROUND

For almost 50 years, Bosnia and Herzegovina was one of the six republics forming the Socialist Federative Republic of Yugoslavia, popularly known as Federal or Second Yugoslavia. The Second Yugoslavia became a reality at the end of the World War II with the Communist seizure of power after the complete obliteration of the first Yugoslavia, known as the Kingdom of Yugoslavia. The first Yugoslavia emerged after World War I as a result of the destruction of the prewar Ottoman and Habsburg empires. Initially, it was called the Kingdom of Serbs, Croats and Slovenes. In 1929, it was renamed as the Kingdom of Yugoslavia (Malcolm, 1994), and lasted for 20 years until it was destroyed physically by the German invasion in 1941 and divided between Germany, Italy, Hungary and Bulgaria.

The Second Yugoslavia was created by Tito's Yugoslav Communist Party (KPJ) but generated and finally shaped as a consequence of Tito's Partisan victory, as well as the ending of the Second World War by the Allied Forces. This Yugoslavia was founded in 1943 in Jajce, during the second assembly of Tito's Anti-Fascist Council of National Liberation of Yugoslavia (Malcolm, 1994). It was described as a state of six republics (Bosnia-Hercegovina, Croatia, Macedonia, Montenegro, Serbia, and Slovenia), five nations, three religions, four languages, two scripts and one goal of living in "brotherhood and unity." Similarly, like the first manifestation, the new Communist Yugoslavia did not last very long, actually surviving for only 46 years. For almost half of that time, from 1968 onwards, it was in a state of decline, finally breaking apart eleven years after the death of Tito, when the two republics of Slovenia and Croatia voted in favor of independence on the 25th and 26th of June 1991, respectively.

The disintegration of Tito's Yugoslavia began with economic decline and the failure of federal leadership, and culminated in deep ethnic crises. The power vacuum after Tito's death opened up possibilities for new leaders in the republics. In 1986, the first new and strong leaders appeared – Milan Kučan in Slovenia and Slobodan Milošević in Serbia. During the late 1980s in Croatia, Franjo Tuđman came into sight. Their different visions of leadership of the Federation led to political disagreements and confrontations, including the breakup of the Federal League of Communists, and eventually of Yugoslavia itself. The illusion of "brotherhood and unity" that was led by Communist indoctrination for years was crushed when Slovenia and Croatia seceded from the Federation, and were almost immediately invaded by Serbia. However, while the independence of Slovenia was formally accepted by Serbian president Milošević after a brief and relatively bloodless ten-day war in which the JNA (Yugoslav National Army) was defeated, Croatia's declaration of independence unleashed ethnic phobias and tensions between Croats and local Serbs supported by the JNA. These tensions turned into a vicious and bloody war in which more than 20,000 people lost their lives (Silber and Little, 1995; Lampe, 2000).

The fate of the third Yugoslav Republic of Bosnia-Hercegovina, a territory surrounded by Croatia, Serbia and Montenegro, and populated by three ethnic groups – Muslims, Croats and Serbs – was doomed from the very moment its government proposed independence through the creation of an independent state of Bosnia and Herzegovina. Immediately after this proposal was floated, on the 9th of January 1992, Bosnian Serbs declared their intention of proclaiming a separate and entirely Serbian territory within the Republic of Bosnia-Hercegovina that would be called the Serb Republic, and would begin functioning if the international community recognised the independence of Bosnia-Hercegovina from the Federal Yugoslavia. Concurrently, the Milošević regime began appealing for ethnic solidarity through a fanatical and paranoid propaganda campaign conducted from Belgrade. The Serbian mass media focused on atrocities committed against Serbs during the Second World War, with the aim of arousing fear in Serbs living outside of Serbia, especially in Bosnia Hercegovina. This succeeded in coercing them to seek protection within a so-called "Greater Serbia," an entity that would extend from north to south, including Kosovo, Montenegro, part of Croatia, and most of the territory of Bosnia-Hercegovina. The only obstacle in establishing Greater Serbia were the Muslims and Croats living within these territories, who would never willingly agree to this, and would therefore have to be eliminated (Cohen, 1998).

On the 29th of February and the 1st of March 1992, a referendum on the independence of Bosnia-Hercegovina was held. Most Bosnian Serbs boycotted the referendum. Of the 64 percent of eligible voters who cast their ballots, 99 percent voted for independence, which was declared two days later on March 3rd 1992. At the same time, Bosnia-Hercegovina, the former, republic of Yugoslavia, changed its name slightly to Bosnia and Herzegovina (BiH).

On the 6th of April 1992, the independence of Bosnia and Herzegovina was recognised by the European Union, and a day later by the United States. Immediately after the EU recognition, the third and by far the cruelest and the bloodiest of the ethnic wars started, one that became the hallmark of Yugoslav disintegration. JNA units composed of Bosnian Serbs began shelling Sarajevo, and at the same time, the "ethnic cleansing" of Muslims and Croats from eastern, northern and northwestern Bosnia commenced. Bosnian Serbs were assisted by armed Serbian paramilitary forces which had crossed the Drina River from Serbia into eastern Bosnia, and who had coincidentally already been involved in the massacring of Muslims in the town of Bijeljina since April 1st (Maass, 1996).

By August 1992, a great part of the country had been "cleansed" of its non-Serbian occupants, and Bosnian Serbs took control of over more than 70 percent of the territory of Bosnia and Herzegovina. Several hundred thousand Muslims and Croats were either killed on the spot, imprisoned in concentration camps, in which most were eventually killed, or driven out from their homes (Vulliamy, 1994).

In April 1993, the political and military leaders of Bosnian Croats, inspired by the international community's plan of dividing the territory of Bosnia and Herzegovina into ten ethnically pure cantons, and supported by Croatian president Franjo Tuđman, announced the creation of the so-called Croatian Republic Herceg-Bosnia. To accomplish their goal of having their own territory populated only by Croats, they began the "ethnic cleansing" of the Muslims populations within central Bosnia and western Herzegovina (Gow, 1997; Burgh and Shoup, 1999).

The war in Bosnia and Herzegovina that began in April 1992 ended with the Dayton negotiations in November 1995. Bosnia and Herzegovina came out of the war with deep wounds, to a great extent destroyed, and divided into two entities: the Federation of BiH (run together by Muslims, now called Bosniaks and Croats) and the Serb Republic administered and largely populated by Serbs.

Ten years after the culmination of this war, the actual numbers of the dead and displaced are still controversial and widely disputed. The number of more than 200,000 dead cited for years was recently lowered to around 100,000 by independent research conducted by the Research and Documentation Centre (Skirbič, 2006), whilst the number of missing persons remains the same – approximately 30,000. Of the majority of all missing persons, about 90 percent were Muslims killed during 1992 and 1993 in ethnic cleansing operations, and in 1995 after the fall of Srebrenica.

EXHUMATION, EXAMINATION AND IDENTIFICATION AS AN INTEGRATED PROCESS IN BiH

The very first exhumations in BiH began in autumn 1995, and were conducted by local authorities who, except for the International Criminal Tribunal for the former Yugoslavia (ICTY), were from the very beginning the only parties responsible for the process of exhumation, examination and identification of missing persons. The main purpose of the exhumations that local Commissions for tracing missing persons representing Croats, Bosniaks (Muslims) and Serbs carried out was, and still is, the identification of recovered remains and the returning of the victims to their families. In early summer 1996, ICTY, the only foreign agency which had the authority to investigate any grave in the territory of the former Yugoslavia, began exhumation activities in order to collect evidence of war crimes committed there during the war of 1991–1995. ICTY forensic teams, comprised of forensic experts from all over the world, carried out exhumations and consequently the examination of recovered remains until 2001, accordingly to the needs and strategy of the ICTY prosecutor's office. The majority of ICTY's activities in Bosnia and Herzegovina were concerned with exhumation of primary and secondary graves, containing the remains of more then 8,000 men from Srebrenica, murdered between the 13th and 17th of July, 1995 in eastern Bosnia, and subsequently buried in countless mass graves. Apart from exhuming the so-called Srebrenica graves, the ICTY forensic team also worked in northern Bosnia, recovering the remains of victims of concentration camps such as Luka in Brcko, and Omarska and Keraterm in the Krajina area. All bodies recovered and examined by the ICTY forensic teams were subsequently transferred into the custody of the Bosniak authorities, who were responsible for their identification. For years the identifications, especially of the fragmented and highly commingled remains of the Srebrenica victims, was an unsolvable and frustrating nightmare.

The only exception to the rule in the control of exhumation activities in BiH by the local authorities and the ICTY occurred in June of 1996. In late spring of 1996, Elisabeth Rehn, a former Finnish defence minister, who in 1996 was a representative of the UN Human Rights Commission in the former Yugoslavia, visited an area in the eastern part of Bosnia close to Srebrenica. She become so deeply upset after seeing hundreds of human remains scattered over the hillsides above the village of Kravica, that she demanded that the remains be collected, identified, and returned to their families. This activity was to be conducted on a humanitarian, not human rights, basis. Her public and very emotional appeal was ignored by the international community; only the Finnish government responded by providing a grant of $500,000 USD, three de-miners and a team of forensic pathologists.

The Finnish team travelled to the region of Kravica without any military escort, and without permission from the authorities of the Serb Republic. On the hills above Kravica, they managed to collect the bones of between 30 and 35 individuals, some clothing, personal artefacts and several identity cards, before they were chased away by the local Serbian police. Such an action, widely criticized by the international community, was never repeated (USIP, 1996). The remains collected by the Finnish team were identified years later with the use of DNA analysis.

During this first year's exhumation "season," from the end of 1995 until the end of 1996, the remains of approximately 2,000 persons were either exhumed from mass graves, or collected from the surface of the ground in fields and forests. The next year brought a significant decline of exhumation activities, especially of so-called "inter-entity" exhumations (exhumations carried out by Bosniak and Croat Commissions in the territory of the Serb Republic or the Serbian Commission in the territory of the Federation). Even the ICTY forensic team did not work in 1997 on the Srebrenica graves, but instead in the town of Brcko, exhuming only 63 bodies.

There were many complex factors, mainly of a political and financial nature, which served to stall the exhumation process during 1997. Finally, in November of that year, due to mutual agreement reached by all three parties (Bosniaks, Croats and Serbs) regarding the rules of conducting so-called "inter-entity" exhumations, as well as a result of some humanitarian donations, the process of conducting exhumations was resumed. In 1998, there was a sharp rise in exhumation activities all across Bosnia and Herzegovina. During that year, most of the exhumations were carried out by Bosniak and Croat Commissions in Herzegovina, in the northwestern region of Bosnia called the Krajina, and in the eastern part of Bosnia, near the town Rogatica. The Serbian Commission was searching for the missing mostly in the Sarajevo area, and in Ozren, a mountainous area close to the town of Tuzla. In the following years until 2006, the remains of thousands of victims were exhumed from several hundred graves.

Exhumation, Examination and Identification

From the very beginning, the whole process of exhumation, post-mortem examination, and identification of recovered mortal remains in Bosnia and Herzegovina was carried out under the legal aegis of BiH government auspices, such as the Courts and Prosecutor Offices of both BiH entities, and involved many persons and institutions.

Since the end of the war until 2003, exhumations had been conducted under the jurisdiction of the relevant Courts, after Commissions for tracing missing persons revealed the locations of sites, and determined the time required for exhumation activities. From 2004, the Prosecutor's Offices took control of the entire process, and prosecutors replaced the so-called "investigative judges."

Every step of the process involves the participation of many individuals representing different institutions and specialities, such as criminal investigators and crime scene technicians, court-appointed forensic pathologists and autopsy technicians, local members of Commissions for tracing missing persons, and locally hired manual labourers (grave diggers, backhoe operators, drivers, etc.) all working together under the jurisdiction of the prosecutor.

From 1997 on, in cases when exhumations had to be conducted in a territory under Serbian administration, the Bosniak and Croat Commissions had to obtain permission for launching exhumation activities from the Office of the High Representative (OHR), which was responsible for executing the Dayton accords on behalf of the international community. This was also applicable if the Serbian Commission wanted to conduct exhumations in the territory of the Federation. Later on, in 2001, the International Commission on Missing Persons (ICMP), established in 1996 to help clarify the fate of the missing persons in the former Yugoslavia, took control of these coordinating responsibilities from OHR. However, if any Commission conducted exhumations in its own territory, there was no need for requesting approval from any international organization, or other party, unless the site was a priority for the ICTY indictments (as were most of the sites containing the remains of victims from Srebrenica, or from various concentration camps).

From the end of 1996 until the end of 2000, the exhumation process was monitored by foreign forensic specialists, such as anthropologists, archaeologists and forensic pathologists. These forensic monitors were provided by two American NGOs, first by Physicians for Human Rights

(PHR), and then by Kenyon International, both financed by ICMP. Some of the PHR and Kenyon monitors took a more active part in the process by assisting local teams with exhumations, but they were very rarely present at examinations, and never took part in identifications.

OHR and IPTF (International Police Task Forces) representatives also monitored the exhumations by observing the activities of the exhumation teams, by recording the names of sites and the number of exhumed remains, while SFOR (Stabilisation Forces in BiH) merely provided security.

In 2001, ICMP took over from OHR, assuming responsibility for monitoring exhumations, as well as actively assisting local authorities in the entire process by providing forensic experts for exhumations and examinations, necessary equipment and supplies. Using recent advances in DNA technology, ICMP introduced a pioneering DNA program on a massive scale as a new strategy for the identification of unknown remains. Since 2002, almost all identifications in Bosnia and Herzegovina have been conducted with the help of DNA.

The exhumation season depends on the weather, and under optimal conditions, can last up to 9 months (from March through November). Exhumations are carried out across Bosnia and Herzegovina (see Fig. 7-1). The majority of the activities were, and still are, concentrated in areas of northwest Bosnia, in the so-called Krajina region (more than 5000 missing), eastern Bosnia (from Srebrenica alone, almost 8400 went missing during July 1995) and in Herzegovina (more then 2000 missing). Since late 1996, exhumations of Bosniaks (Muslims) killed during the war between 1992 and 1995, were coordinated by members of the State Commission for Tracing Missing Persons. The Commission was established in April 1992 as the Commission for Exchange of POWs, and for the next four years, its members were busy dealing with the exchange of prisoners of war, in addition to the remains of those who were killed. After the war, the Commission changed its name to the State Commission for Tracing Missing Persons, and acted under the patronage and financial support of the Ministry of Justice of the Federation of BiH. During early 1999, the financial status quo of the Commission became more than uncertain, and it began to depend heavily on donations from the ICMP. Actually, from the beginning, all three Commissions in BiH had some support from the international community, either in the form of money, or in donations of equipment or basic supplies, such as body bags, protective overalls, gloves, etc. Usually all do-

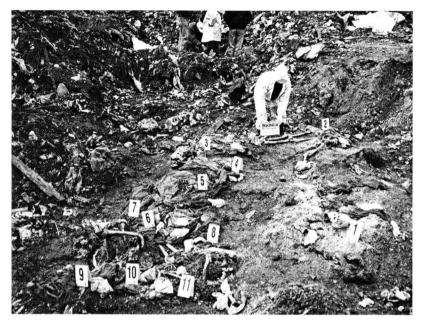

Figure 7-1. Mass grave at garbage dump in Ivan Polje. Exhumation conducted
in September 2000.

nations were distributed equally between the three parties involved in
the process of exhuming missing persons, unless it was an exclusive
one-party donation, such as the British government's donation to the
Serbian Commission in 1997. Unfortunately, such donations have never
been sufficient and/or sustained, especially for the Bosniaks, whose
people counted for approximately 90 percent of all missing persons.

The State Commission for Tracing Missing Persons did not possess
any legal powers, except for that of influence through the respect and
admiration for its activities, and especially for its president. During
2000, under pressure from the international community represented by
the Office of the High Representative (OHR), the Bosniak and Croat
Commissions merged into one body and became the Federation Commission on Missing Persons.

In BiH, like everywhere else, the responsibilities of all governmental
structures are clearly defined by law, and the police are in charge of collecting information about missing persons. However, during and after
the war, with most of the country's structures destroyed, and the sheer
amount of people unaccounted for, families were reporting information
about the missing to the closest available authority. In some areas in

which the Commission did not have a representative, the police were responsible for the registration of missing persons, while in others, members of the Commission registered that information. Regardless of who took the information, both parties cooperated closely.

From the very beginning, the process of exhumation and identification was plagued by a notorious lack of sufficient funds, basic necessary equipment and supplies, and a deficiency of qualified forensic experts, such as forensic pathologists, anthropologists or archaeologists. Since nobody was really prepared by any means for such an enormous task of exhuming, examining and identifying a seemingly innumerable amount of remains from the start, the approach taken toward exhumations was very often extremely unprofessional. With no local anthropologists and archaeologists, and with very few forensic pathologists in Bosnia and Herzegovina, exhumations were often carried out merely by untrained workers and Commission members. Unfortunately, in many situations, basic lack of knowledge, egos, ignorance and politics ruled over principal best practice activities. Identifications were accomplished in the traditional and only manner possible in those days, that being through the recognition of clothing and personal artefacts by surviving family members.

A donation by the Icelandic government enabled this author, a forensic anthropologist, to work on the exhumation, examination and identification process with the Bosniak State Commission for Tracing Missing Persons between 1998 and 2000. Experiences from this period are presented in the following section.

General Activities on the Ground – Theory and Practice

The main activity of the Bosniak Commission members was, and still is, collecting information pertaining to missing persons, and searching for burial sites and clandestine mass graves. In general, there are six major geographic areas in which the Bosniak Commission has been working on exhumations since late 1995. They are: Krajina in northwestern Bosnia, the western part of Herzegovina, central Bosnia, Podrinje in eastern Bosnia (where apart from other graves are all of the graves containing the victims of Srebrenica), southeastern Bosnia around the towns of Rogatica and Višegrad, and southern Bosnia around the towns of Gorazde and Foca. Before exhumations could be conducted, members of the Commission had to check every piece of information about the location of grave(s) reported to them, which is accomplished during so-called "pre-visits." In the first years after the war, these investigative visits were carried out by the Commission members alone, or in the company of informants who were either survivors of the massacres, or eyewitnesses to the executions. Very often, those people were not only frightened to go back to areas where the killings took place, but were also terrified that they might be recognised by perpetrators while travelling into remote locations, deep into the territories that once were their homes, but that after the war became part of the Serb Republic. Since the Commission did not have vehicles with protective windows, the OHR came forward, providing their own cars and monitors, which provided the necessary security to witnesses.

After grave locations were established, and all parties taking part in the process of exhumation agreed with proposed dates, the exhumations could then commence. As a mode of practice, the Commission member responsible for the process in his/her area of operation informed the investigative judge assigned by Cantonal Court about the existence of graves, and about the expected amount of time that exhumation activities would take. The judge then officially notified other members of a so-called "team of experts" such as court-appointed forensic pathologists and autopsy technicians, criminal investigators and crime scene technicians, as well as a funeral company, seconding digging equipment, backhoe operators and manual labourers, while the commission member would usually coordinate future activities according to the schedule of all participants. During the dates on which the exhumations were scheduled, all members of the expert team, as well as other participants, gathered at a designated meeting place. If the exhumations were to be carried out in the territory of the Serb Republic, the meeting place was on the so-called "line of separation," an invisible border separating Bosnia and Herzegovina (according to the Dayton agreement) into two entities, the Federation of BiH and the Serb Republic, where a convoy of cars carrying the exhumation team and accompanying persons was formed. Apart from the members of the exhumation team, there were always local representatives of Serbian authorities present such as members of the Serbian Commission, crime scene technicians, local police providing escort, in addition to international monitors, and very often, mass media representatives.

During these first years of exhumations, the daily routine began with checking the list of names of all participants. Usually the procedure of verification of names and other formalities was performed smoothly, and the convoy could then drive to the location, or locations, designated for that day. However, from time to time, the Serbs had some objections. One day they might claim that the list contained the names of the "war criminals" while on another, that there were "too many names." Frequently, their objections caused long and emotional discussions that eventually had to be terminated with help of the accompanying monitors representing the international community (OHR).

The majority of the locations opened at the very beginning of exhumations in 1998 were single or multiple graves, situated in close proximity to ruined houses in completely destroyed villages, in surrounding fields, or nearby forests. On a daily basis, the exhumation team moved from one location to another, attempting to open all the graves scheduled for each day, and fulfil the expectations of surviving family members for the recovery of their loved ones' remains. Since there were hundreds of sites to be opened, and the exhumation period heavily limited by the Cantonal Courts' funds, the members of the Commission tried to schedule work with as many graves as they thought possible to open and exhume on each day. Such restrictions led to situations in which exhumations were conducted hastily, and the people working on the recovery process were frequently and persistently reminded to speed up digging, cleaning and recovering remains, because other sites were waiting for them to open. Additional problems were caused by the lack of forensically trained experts. In the first years after the war, there were only six forensic pathologists working in Bosnia and Herzegovina, with four more in training, but none of them were really adequately trained or prepared for the task of exhuming hundreds of graves, containing thousands of victims of war, nor did they have enough time to spend in the field on exhumations. In addition to these challenges, there was not a single local anthropologist or archaeologist present in Bosnia and Herzegovina to assist with exhumations and identifications. Consequently, more often than not, exhumations were carried out in a very unprofessional way, due to the lack of experts, the lack of basic knowledge held by people working on recovery, the egos of team members, or because of conflicting political agendas.

During March of 1997, the author, under the patronage of PHR, organised several training courses presenting exhumation, examination and identification issues. The courses were given to the representatives of local authorities (pathologists, autopsy technicians, crime investigators and crime scene technicians, judges and prosecutors), as well as to the members of the three Commissions involved in tracing missing persons, dealing with the process of exhumation, examination and identification of victims of the past war. The courses were supplemented with a manual specially written for this occasion and published in Serbo-Croatian (Klonowski, 1997).

In spite of this, the exhumation practices often had very little in common with the theory on how to open and exhume graves as taught on these courses. On the other hand, the theory as conveyed in the courses had very little in common with the dreadful realities with which the local Bosnian exhumation teams had to cope during the early days of exhumation activities.

At that time, in general, exhumations were conducted in a hostile environment, within remote and unpopulated territories often still controlled by the perpetrators. Security measures, such as presence of the SFOR forces, were rarely provided, while mine assessment was hardly ever available. With the country's economy barely able to keep its inhabitants going, there was a chronic shortage of basic supplies, necessary equipment, and transportation.

The author describes typical exhumation day in her notes from July 1998:

> The first three locations today were situated close to each other – just several hundred meters apart. The first place was situated close to the village's main road in something that once was an orchard. Six years ago, on 23 July 1992, the witness buried here his mother, wife and two small children killed by Serbian paramilitary troopers. He memorised the place, which he covered with some branches. When the first exhumation season began, he showed the site to the Commission representative.
>
> After the crime scene technician took the photographs of the site the workers set off with their usual routine of cleaning the place of the grass and six years' overgrowth of bushes and next began to dig the first trench. Since the soil was very dry, compact and stone hard, manual unearthing the top layer of the grave had to take quite a while. To save time needed for opening two other sites, the team was divided into three groups. At the first location an autopsy technician was left to supervise digging. The second location, a mass grave with the bodies of five men, family members of another witness, was down the steep slope on the bottom of the hill, in a wet field covered with tall grass and surrounded by a grove of trees. Again, the crime scene technician took photographs of the site and the workers began digging a first trench. The opening of

this site was under the author's supervision. A local pathologist with the rest of the workers took care of the third site, a single grave located a little bit farther up on a hill.

The first trench at the author's site was dug in the wrong place – the soil was getting more compact when the labourers dug deeper. The second trench, a couple of metres away from the first one, was in the right place and soon after excavation began a shoe was exposed. After the borders of the grave were established, the workers began carefully removing the top soil until they reached a thick plastic sheet covering all the bodies. The bodies were very well preserved, in the state of saponification. They were placed in two layers – three bodies on the bottom and two on top of them. After the photographs were taken of the bodies, one after another one was delineated, lifted from the grave, and placed into marked body bags. After all bodies were removed, the bottom of the grave was carefully checked. In the meantime the third team finished exhuming the single grave and all members of the team joined labourers and the autopsy technician working at the first location. Finally, the hard covering layer of the soil was removed and a blanket and leather jacket covering remains was exposed. Both the jacket (belonging to the witness) and the blanket were carefully pulled off, exposing two tiny skeletons that were placed on top of another blanket which covered two adult skeletons. After photographs were taken, the forensic pathologist, the author, and the autopsy technician began separating and collecting tiny bones comprising skeletons. The bones of the little boy were collected together with partially preserved shorts and his small sandals. Subsequently, after all the bones were collected it was possible to lift the blanket up exposing two female skeletons. Then the same procedure proceeded – placing the numbers, taking photographs, and collecting all bones into separate body bags.

With three more locations that day, there was no lunch break – everybody ate in the cars, on the way to other locations. Again, there were three locations relatively close to each other. The first one was nearby an old and abandoned Muslim graveyard. The third witness that day, a young woman, pointed out two graves. One was a single grave and one a mass grave with nine bodies that were her closest family members. The last, third grave, also a single one, was situated down the slope, at the bottom of the hill, by a row of trees and bushes. After the photographs were taken, the sites were cleaned of bush and the workers began digging. The two single graves were dug up in an hour while digging up the third, bigger one took much more time due to the fact that the soil was again very compact and hard. With all trenches around the burial completed, the author, forensic pathologist and autopsy technician began removing the last layer of soil with trowels and after another hour they exposed skeletons. Since it was already getting late, some workers helped in final cleaning, as well as one of the PHR monitors. Even the witness helped by passing plastic bags used for collecting hand and foot bones as requested by team members. Anyhow, it took an additional hour more to completely expose all nine skeletons. One was wrapped in a blanket, two covered by another blanket; six lay side-by-side, not covered by anything and with the bones of their arms and legs commingled. After the photographs were taken the remains were carefully separated and then collected into marked body bags. The bottom of the pit was checked out, grave filled back with the soil, and the long work day was over at half-past seven. Remains of 21 people were exhumed which was a kind of record. Yesterday 16 bodies were dug up in the forest.

Quoted above, the author's original notes describe one of the better exhumation days. Despite very high temperatures, the lack of a backhoe, difficulties with manual digging, and the great number of remains that had to be exhumed that day, there was no usual rush, and the exhumations were carried out in a quite professional manner.

Unfortunately, there were also days when everything went wrong, often starting with arguments at the meeting point on the line of separation. Then the first gravesite could not be located and the judge and the Commission representative would argue about the credibility of the informant. With time passing mercilessly by because of fruitless searching, the judge would decide to drive to the next location. Then the pathologist would get into a foul mood because he would feel that his position was being intimidated by the presence of a volunteering anthropologist (the author) and monitoring pathologist (representing PHR) and he would threaten to leave the exhumation site if "the foreigners" would be working on it. To solve the problem, the Commission representative and judge would resign themselves to the pathologist's requests, and exhumations would be carried out by unskilled workers with the pathologist ordering that the collections of bones, which were scattered in the grass and inside the destroyed summer house, were to be placed randomly into several body bags. All other sites that day would be exhumed in a similar way, by workers. The very long day would end in the late evening with the pathologist demonstratively leaving the last site due to the fact that the Commission representative would not listen to his suggestion to quit the work because of the late hour, and leaving behind the already exposed remains in the process (Klonowski, 1999).

The exhumations in Bosnia and Herzegovina, which local authorities carry out, began first of all for humanitarian purposes, whilst collecting evidence of the committed crimes, work that the local crime investigators and crime scene technicians are responsible for, is an important additional activity. On a practical level, this task is in the hands of persons working in the graves who are reporting the discovery of cartridges, bullets, documents or other artefacts, presenting these to onsite crime investigators and crime scene technicians, who would then take photographs and document the findings.

Each exhumation is followed by the second step of the exhumation and identification process, which is the examination of recovered remains (see Fig.7-2). Similar to the exhumation process, the examination

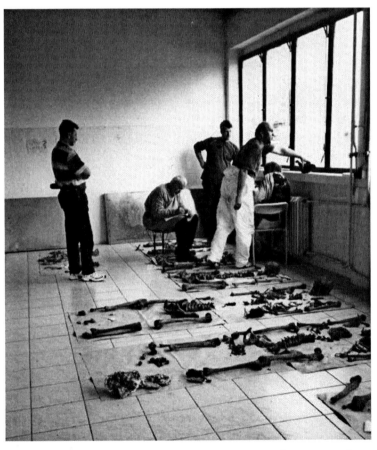

Figure 7-2. Forensic pathologist and crime scene technicians working on examination at Sanski Most.

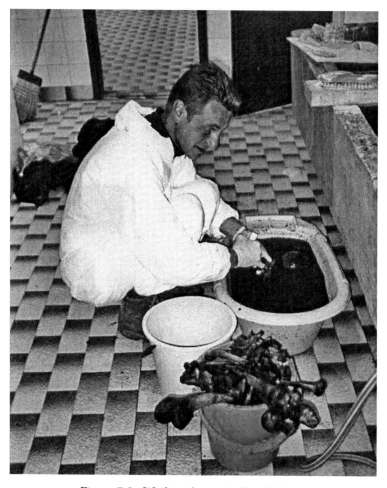

Figure 7-3. Washing bones in Sanski Most.

approach was notoriously unprofessional, showing a lack of basic standard procedures and scientific methodology. For years, neither remains nor clothing were washed before examination (see Fig. 7-3). In some regions, the examination was conducted by the autopsy technician, who reported his findings to the pathologist who was taking notes. Both forensic pathologists and autopsy technicians did not have practice in examining skeletonised remains, as well as not being aware of any methods of assessing age, except that of cranial suture fusion. Eventually, with time passing by, some pathologists began using standard aging methods and other examination techniques that were introduced in the courses in 1997, while others were happy to use the help of the author

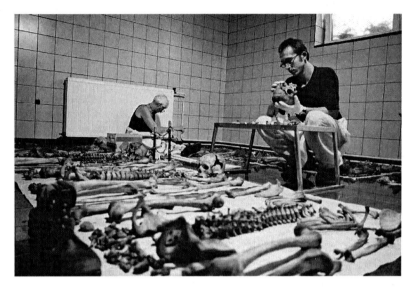

Figure 7-4. Anthropologists working in Visoko's morgue.

on a volunteering basis (see Fig. 7-4). Unfortunately, there were also those who were neither prepared to accept new methods nor the anthropologist's help, and whose autopsy reports were frequently marred with mistakes and incorrect conclusions.

Identification Process

At its inception, the identification process was held simultaneously with the examination. In some areas, families were allowed and encouraged to participate in identifications before the postmortem examinations were finished. The identifications were performed in a very traditional and only possible way in those days, that being by the recognition of clothing, personal artefacts, documents, etc. In some cases, however rarely, dental status or old healed injuries were recalled by close family members, these serving to play an additional role in the identification of the remains. However, the majority of such information could not be supported by any records, due to the fact that most medical and dental records were destroyed during the war.

In some locations, family members present at the examination would attempt, together with the examining pathologist, to confirm information provided on the spot by the pathologist, and if the antemortem data was confirmed by postmortem findings, the identification documents could be signed and remains immediately released. Such practices would not allow other families the possibility to see the clothing pertaining to the recovered remains. Taking into consideration the fact that recovered garments were not washed, and that the victim wearing recognised clothing was seen last quite a long time ago, there was always a risk that the identification would be incorrect. There were also situations in which two different families claimed the same remains because of recognition of familiar clothing or shoes, while antemortem information was poor, and insufficient enough for a definitive conclusion as to which family could sign the identification documents. In such circumstances, and with no other means to assist in the identification, the process turned into arguments that eventually had to be settled in arbitration by the judge.

Given the sheer number of exhumed mortal remains, and with many of those exhumed from mass graves being deteriorated and unrecognizable, accurate identifications using traditional techniques were often, not surprisingly, almost impossible. Many unidentified victims had to be reinterred as NN (no name) because it was not possible to accurately identify them without the use of DNA.

Eventually, the DNA testing supporting identification process was introduced in 2000 by the ICMP. This served to establish a unique pioneering program, which led to the positive identifications of unknown remains based on the comparison of DNA profiles obtained from bone samples of exhumed human remains, in conjunction with DNA profiles of blood samples from the missing persons' relatives. Thanks to this program, the first positive DNA match to identify unknown remains of a young Srebrenica victim was obtained in November 2001. As of July 2006, the ICMP' DNA laboratories have generated DNA matches for more than 8,000 missing persons in Bosnia and Herzegovina.

SUMMARY

The exhumation and identification process carried out in Bosnia and Herzegovina is an organised unique activity, conducted under the aegis and financial sponsorship of the BiH government for humanitarian purposes. At the end of the 1992–1995 war, approximately 30,000 persons were unaccounted for, and listed as missing. Immediately after the conclusion of the war, three local governmental Commissions for tracing missing persons were organised to search for graves, and to exhume the mortal remains of reported missing persons (Bosniaks, Croats and Serbs). A couple of years later, the Bosniak and Croat Commissions merged into one that was named the Federal Commission for Tracing Missing Persons, whilst the Serb Commission stayed unchanged, and remained a separate entity. As a result of years of activities, the remains of about 15,000 persons have been exhumed from thousands of single and multiple graves, and about 400 mass graves.

During the initial years, the exhumation and examination process was plagued by a notorious lack of money, supplies, qualified staff, basic security, and a dreadful political situation. Traditional methods of identification, relying on the recognition of clothing and personal artefacts were used for establishing the identity of unknown human remains. If recognition of those items was supported by positive results of post-mortem and antemortem comparisons of the individual's features such as sex, age, stature and dental status, the remains were declared as identified, and released to family members. With the lack of more sophisticated methods, this procedure was widely used across Bosnia and Herzegovina, especially pertaining to the identifications of victims buried soon after death in single or multiple graves, these being conducted by surviving family members or neighbours. Traditional methods failed when confronted with the identification of victims recovered from mass graves, both primary and secondary. The huge numbers of individuals, the degraded state of remains representing victims of a similar age, mostly male, combined with a lack of sufficiently detailed medical and dental records, reduced the effectiveness of traditional identification. This situation has changed significantly since 2001, with the introduction of DNA-led methods of identification. Since then, more than 8,000 remains have been positively identified with utilization of DNA analysis.

REFERENCE

Burgh, S.L., and Shoup, P.S. (1999). *The war in Bosnia-Herzegovina, ethnic conflict and international intervention.* Armonk, N.N.: M.E. Sharpe.
Cohen, R. (1998). Chronology. In: *Hearts grown brutal: Sagas of Sarajevo.* New York: Random House.
Gow, J. (1997). *The triumph of the lack of will, international diplomacy and the Yugoslav war.* New York: Columbia University Press.

Klonowski, E. (1997). *Priručnik. Uputstva za ekshumaciju i identifikaciju ljudskog skeleta.* PHR. GIK "OKO" Sarajevo.

Klonowski, E. (1999). *Exhumations in Godinske Bare on 28 April 1999.* Report.

Klonowski, E. (2007). Exhumations in Bosnia and Herzegovina: Caves as mass graves, from recovery to identification. In *Forensic anthropology: Case studies from Europe,* Brickley, M., and Ferllini, R. (Eds.). Springfield: Charles C Thomas. In press.

Lampe, J.R. (2000). *Yugoslavia as history: Twice there was a country.* Cambridge: Cambridge University Press.

Maass, P. (1996). *Love thy neighbour: A story of war.* New York: Alfred A. Knopf, Inc.

Madajczyk, C. (1989). *Dramat Katyński.* Warszawa: Ksiazka i Wiedza.

Malcolm, N. (1994). *Bosnia: A short history.* London: Macmillan.

Paul, A. (1991). *Katyń. Stalins's massacre and the seeds of Polish resurrection.* Annapolis: Charles Scribner's Sons, Naval Institute Press.

Silber, L., and Little, A. (1995). *Yugoslavia: Death of a nation.* London: Penguin Books.

Skirbič, M. (2006). *Counting the dead: New research into the number of war dead proves divisive.* http://www.tol.cz/look/TOL/article.tpl?IdLanguage=1&IdPublication=4&NrIssue=161&NrSection=1&NrArticle=16246 Accessed 8 August 2006.

US Institute of Peace (USIP)(1996). *Mass graves and exhumations.* Sarajevo: Department of Human Rights and Refugees, Office of the High Representative.

Vulliamy, E. (1994). *Season's in hell: Understanding Bosnia's war.* London: Simon & Schuster, Ltd.

Chapter 8

WHO IS MISSING?
PROBLEMS IN THE APPLICATION
OF FORENSIC ARCHAEOLOGY
AND ANTHROPOLOGY
IN COLOMBIA'S CONFLICT

Ana María Gómez López and Andrés Patiño Umaña

INTRODUCTION

Forensic archaeology is the application of archaeological techniques to the recovery of evidence and human remains in judicial contexts. Forensic anthropology, as a sister discipline, focuses on the analysis of human remains using biological anthropology. Human remains can be buried or hidden in a variety of circumstances, and forensic archaeologists and anthropologists are regularly employed to recover and analyze remains in order to investigate such deaths for legal and humanitarian purposes. Such deaths may range from domestic criminal cases to international human rights investigations. In the last decade, the forensic investigation of mass graves has been on the rise (Haglund, 2002:244). These international investigations of human rights violations and crimes against humanity worldwide have benefited from the participation of forensic archaeologists (Haglund, 2002; Juhl, 2005) and forensic anthropologists (Burns, 1998; Ferllini, 1999; Fondebrider and Doretti, 2001; Steadman and Haglund, 2005).

In Colombia, with particular reference to investigations of disappeared individuals related to the country's ongoing political conflict, forensic archaeologists and anthropologists have the obligation of recovering all finds from mass graves in order to reconstruct what occurred, and to identify the human remains in question. Yet, achieving both of these related goals proves to be difficult when it is not clear who is missing in Colombia. There are currently no exact figures on how many individuals have disappeared due to the country's conflict. This chapter will reflect on the use of forensic archaeology and anthropology in achieving these joint goals in Colombia, focusing on the challenges of locating clandestine cemeteries, and consequently, locating the disappeared. The authors will describe the different scenarios and obstacles encountered, as regularly posed by Colombian armed groups, with particular emphasis on the occurrence of unique clandestine graves in Colombia. Shortfalls of the Colombian authorities in tackling these different settings will be highlighted, in addition to suggestions on how these investigations can be improved. Finally, this chapter will shed light on the humanitarian needs of the victims' families in Colombia, by providing relatives with information and the remains of their loved ones in order to affect closure.

DISAPPEARANCES IN COLOMBIA'S CONFLICT

Colombia is caught in a protracted internal armed conflict. Despite changing manifestations, there has been a historical continuity to Colombia's violence, in which several geographic areas of the country have experienced ongoing conflict, perpetrated by official and illegal armed groups for at least five decades (Chernick, 2003:186). The Colombian state has traditionally been unable to protect the country's civilian population, particularly in rural areas, where governmental institutions have limited reach or presence. Such lawless zones have permitted armed groups to flourish over rival state forces, and exercise strong territorial control (Fig. 8-1).

Currently, Colombia's conflict is characterized by an alarming number of violations of international humanitarian law. Left-wing guerrillas, right-wing paramilitaries, and official security forces, regularly commit atrocious acts of violence toward Colombia's civilian population. Confrontation between these armed groups is rare, and most victims are not killed in the crossfire, but due to direct attacks. Such attacks are motivated by the need for territorial control, during which armed parties will target social activists and community leaders, and will predominantly attack unarmed civilians accused of collaborating with, or belonging to,

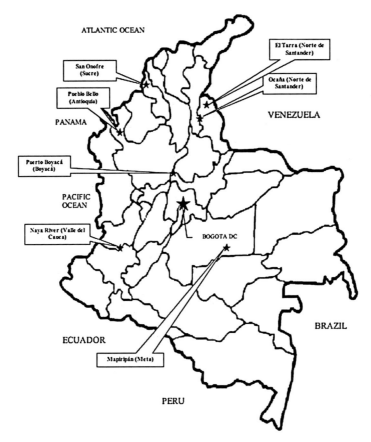

Figure 8-1. Map of Colombia, highlighting areas of interest.

an enemy group. Individuals from marginalized Colombian communities, composed of Afro-Colombian, indigenous and peasant populations, bear the brunt of the country's violence, which has left in its wake almost three million displaced individuals, with hundreds of thousands more dead or "disappeared."

Disappearances[1] are one of the most serious violations of international humanitarian law in Colombia. Scores of individuals are missing

---

1. "Disappearances" are defined by the Colombian Criminal Code as a crime committed by any armed actor. This definition is more wide-reaching than that found in international human rights legislation, but falls under the definition of "missing in conflict," found in the 1949 Geneva Conventions, particularly in Additional Protocol II relating to the Protection of Victims of Non-International Armed Conflicts. For the purposes of this chapter, disappearances will be understood in light of the definition provided by international humanitarian law, which the authors believe is inclusive, and not mutually exclusive, of a strict human rights definition.

in areas controlled by the country's armed factions (Fig. 8-2). While there are no exact figures on the number of the disappeared due to the Colombian conflict, international entities have regularly identified Colombia as a "hot spot" for disappearances worldwide. "The Missing" Project of the International Committee of the Red Cross (ICRC), an initiative which sets guidelines for the treatment of the problem of disappearances worldwide, has denounced disappearances as a practice regularly used to intimidate civilians by all parties in Colombia's conflict (ICRC, 2005). Colombia is also a priority country for the UN Working Group on Enforced or Involuntary Disappearances (UN-WGEID), which has stated in a recent report that, despite substantial underreporting of disappearance cases in Colombia, the situation is still alarming (UNWGEID, 2006).

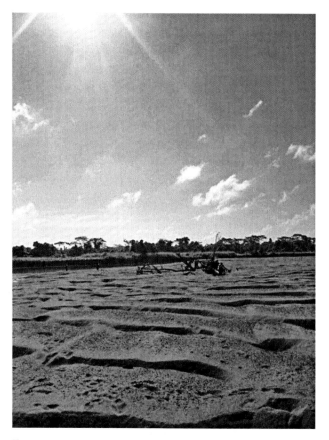

Figure 8-2. Riverbank in northwestern Colombia, where mass graves may be found. Credit: EQUITAS.

DIFFERENT DISPOSAL AND CONCEALMENT PATTERNS BY COLOMBIAN ARMED ACTORS

The *modus operandi* of disappearances by Colombian armed actors makes archaeological recovery and anthropological analyses of human remains extremely difficult. Aside from committing disappearances and selective killings, many groups will go to elaborate lengths with regard to the disposal of the remains of their victims. This involves mutilating and dismembering human remains to ease their concealment, discarding remains in places of difficult access, or resorting to specific burial patterns, as has been observed in other international contexts.[2] Each of these scenarios poses specific logistical difficulties for Colombian judicial investigators, creating contexts which require "flexible excavation strategies" (Hoshower, 1998). The identification of these methods of body dismemberment and disposal by Colombian-armed factions can provide valuable information with regard to the particular group involved in the crime, attempts made to hide evidence of the crime committed, or the given time period during which a disposal location was utilized.

Despite a large body of testimonial evidence of the practices described below, there are very few academic studies that refer to these concealment patterns in Colombia. Most descriptions of such practices are available in national and international non-governmental reports.[3] Many of these practices are not documented in scientific peer-reviewed publications. This chapter constitutes the first attempt to scientifically approach these patterns as typologies, and is meant to be a starting

---

2. Such patterns of concealment are recognized by the United Nations in its *Report of the Secretary-General on human rights and forensic sciences submitted pursuant to Commission on Human Rights, Resolution 1992/24:* "Aside from the political and practical reasons involved, adequate investigations may also be precluded by the fact that the bodies have been disposed of in a manner that prevents their use as evidence. For instance, bodies are sometimes burnt, thrown into rivers or seas or buried in shallow pits without any identification; they are sometimes blasted and the remains covered with soil or left uncovered as intimidating evidence of violence. In other cases, the killers deliberately mutilate the body before or after death, to thwart identification or to intimidate others." See E/CN.4/1993/20, February 5, 1993, Introduction, Paragraph 3.

3. In its report about its mission to Colombia, the UN Working Group on Enforced and Involuntary Disappearances stated that "the practice of killing disappeared persons and cutting up or mutilating their bodies, then burying them in individual or mass graves, was reported to be part of the strategy used by perpetrators in attempting to cover up evidence." See UNWGEID 2006, IV D, Paragraph 52.

point for academic discussions on such practices within the national and international scientific community. The examples used to illustrate these patterns are by no means a comprehensive record, but a selective sample that is representative of the practices described below.

Dismemberment

Dismemberment is a common technique regularly attributed to Colombian-armed groups, particularly paramilitary forces. Victims are regularly mutilated, decapitated and dismembered prior to their disposal, often with the use of machetes and chain saws. Often, it is unclear if these acts were committed during, or after the person's death. This gruesome method serves a twofold purpose, both as a form of torture and a concealment mechanism. In the former, dismemberment is a method of terror and a climate of fear among rural populations. For the latter, dismemberment allows for the ready disposal of remains in burial and non-burial contexts.

There are many witness testimonies of victim dismemberment in Colombia, some of which will be described later on. However, there are currently no published studies on perpetrator dismemberment patterns in this country.[4] Colombian judicial institutions do not record such patterns of dismemberment – it often rests on the initiative of individual official investigators to analyze this aspect of violence.[5] Future anthropological analysis of mutilation and dismemberment patterns in recovered osteological material will prove useful in tracking perpetrators, understanding the circumstances of death of the victims, as well as compiling case studies that take into account contextual taphonomic assessments of these remains (Reichs, 1998; Symes et al., 2002).

---

4. These patterns have been, however, the subject of historical and socio-cultural anthropological analyses. See MV Uribe, 2004, Dismembering and expelling: Semantics of political terror in Colombia, *Public Culture*, (16)1, pp. 79–95; and MV Uribe, 2005, *Antropología de la Inhumanidad: Un Ensayo Interpretativo sobre el Terror en Colombia*, Bogotá: Editorial Norma.

5. An excellent preliminary study on paramilitary perpetrator dismemberment and concealment patterns was presented by O Hidalgo, A Díaz and J Castro at the III Latin American Forensic Anthropology Congress, Bogotá, September 2005, in a paper entitled "Sacando Muertos: Aproximación arqueológica y antropológica forense del paramilitarismo en tres zonas de influencia en Colombia."

Non-burial Methods: Disposal of Remains
in Rivers, Ravines and Chasms

There are numerous reports of cases in which Colombian-armed factions have disposed of remains in areas inaccessible to judicial investigators. These non-burial methods of concealing human remains take advantage of Colombia's natural geographic features, as opposed to creating man-made burial sites. All such factors pose demanding professional challenges to judicial investigators, some of which have been explored in other countries in more depth.[6]

Rivers are a frequent location in which remains are reportedly thrown, as has been reported with reference to several of Colombia's large rivers, such as the Cauca and Magdalena. Two cases where this has been evident have received rulings by the Inter-American Court of Human Rights. One concerns the death of 19 merchants who disappeared in 1987, while in the hands of paramilitaries commanded by Henry Pérez in the outskirts of Puerto Boyacá, province of Boyacá. In this case, the dismembered remains of the victims were thrown by the paramilitaries into a tributary that flows into the Magdalena River.[7] The other case relates to the 1997 massacre of 49 inhabitants from the town of Mapiripán, who were tortured, dismembered, disemboweled, decapitated, and thrown into the Guaviare River by members of the United Self-Defense Forces of Colombia (AUC).[8]

Ravines and chasms are also locations used by Colombian-armed factions in order to dispose of human remains. An example of a well-

---

6. *The Final Report of the United Nations Commission of Experts established pursuant to Security Council resolution 780* provides an excellent account of the kind of mass graves that were created in Bosnia Herzegovina and Croatia due to the conflict in the former Yugoslavia. The Report identifies the two same kind of non-burial patterns identified in the Colombian context, the first being "a pattern whereby perpetrators dispose of bodies in pre-existing but non-traditional sites, which provide a ready-made place for body disposal without the use of mechanical diggers or excavators" such as "mineshafts, canals, quarries, landfills, caves and the like" and the second being "a variety of ways which do not embrace actual interment in a grave, be it real or makeshift," where "the most common non-burial method of disposal is the dumping of bodies into rivers." See UN Doc S/1994/674/Add.2 (Vol. V), December 28, 1994. Annex X Mass graves, II, A.

7. Corte Interamericana de Derechos Humanos. Sentencia *Caso 19 Comerciantes vs. Colombia*, July 5, 2004, paragraph 85f.

8. Corte Interamericana de Derechos Humanos. Sentencia *Caso de la Masacre de Mapiripán vs. Colombia*, September 15, 2005, paragraph 96.39.

documented case is the 2001 Naya massacre,[9] in which the United Self-Defense Forces of Colombia (AUC) conducted a killing spree along the Naya River, an isolated area between the provinces of Valle del Cauca and Cauca. The assassinations, which took place during Holy Week, targeted members of several indigenous and Afro-Colombian rural communities located along the Naya River area.[10] Some of the remains of these individuals were allegedly thrown into nearby abysses.[11] Another example in which remains were thrown into a river is that of Javier Francisco Montoya, a Colombian priest who was kidnapped and killed by the Revolutionary Armed Forces of Colombia (FARC-EP) in 2004. His body was found in early May, 2006, in a river mouth in the department of Chocó, close to the Colombian-Panamanian border.[12]

Javier Francisco Montoya's case is representative of many other kidnapping victims who were killed in captivity, and whose remains were disposed of. There are reports of body disposal by Colombian-armed factions in places such as natural chasms, known informally as *botaderos* or "dumps." This is particularly true of kidnapped individuals – it is common for armed factions not only to bury the body of a kidnapped person that dies while in captivity, but to dispose of it in areas that are difficult for recovery by the authorities. An illustrative example is that of Bernardo Vélez White, brother of Colombia's current secretary of education Cecilia Vélez White, who was also kidnapped by the Revolutionary Armed Forces of Colombia (FARC-EP) in 2001. His body was abandoned in the aforementioned conditions, and discovered in 2004 near the township of Cañas Gordas, department of Antioquia.[13] The body

---

9. For more information, please refer to the article by Scott Wilson, "Colombian massacre large, brutal," *The Washington Post*, April 21, 2001. See also T. Christian Miller, "Paramilitaries took no prisoners on the banks of the Naya River," *Los Angeles Times*, May 20, 2001.

10. *Resolución Defensorial No. 009: Sobre la situación de orden público en la región del rio Naya.* Eduardo Cifuentes Muñoz, *Defensor del Pueblo* (Public Ombudsman), Santafé de Bogotá, May 9, 2001.

11. For more information, please refer to "Terror en el Naya," *El País* [Regional newspaper – Cali], April 16, 2001.

12. For more information, please refer to the article "FARC accused over murdered priest," *BBC News*, December 24, 2004 and "Hallan restos de sacerdote secuestrado y fusilado por las FARC," *El Tiempo* [Colombian national newspaper], May 2, 2006. See also UN Office of the High Commissioner for Human Rights in Colombia, Press release, "Condena por el asesinato del padre Javier Francisco Montoya," December 24, 2004. Available at <www.hchr.org.co>

13. For more information, please refer to the article "Colombian rebels kill minister's brother," *The Guardian,* July 9, 2004. See also UN Office of the High Commissioner for Human Rights in Colombia, Press release, "Condena por el asesinato de Bernardo Vélez White," July 9, 2004. Available at <www.hchr.org.co>

was inside a bag, and exhibited signs of torture and a bullet wound to the head.

In many cases of non-burial body disposal, Colombian judicial officials have often failed to locate, or only succeed in partially recovering, the remains of missing individuals. In order to do so as completely as possible, a variety of methods will need to be applied to recover such remains from these difficult contexts. In the cases of rivers, these methods will range from the archaeological survey of riverbanks[14] to searching within the riverbed (see Figure 8-2), taking into account the hydrological characteristics of the river (depth and current speed) that will determine fluvial transport of remains, such as crania (Nawrocki et al., 1997; Bassett and Manheim, 2002). Ravines and chasms will also require equally special methodological approaches. Recovery experiences in other geomorphic microenvironments, such as caves, may be relevant for comparable logistical planning and taphonomic processes that have taken place (Simmons, 2002).

Burial Methods: Remains Disposed in Clandestine Cemeteries

For decades, Colombian armed factions have regularly deposited the remains of their victims in mass graves[15] throughout the country. As is the case with all mass graves, those in Colombia present special challenges for judicial investigators. The presence of multiple, commingled remains make for demanding recovery and tasks; additionally, the analysis of contextual evidence can provide information on events which have transpired (Haglund, 2002; Haglund et al., 2001; Hunter and Cox, 2005; Schmitt, 2002).

However, there is an additional characteristic of mass graves produced in Colombia that leads to unique difficulties in this context; the remains

---

14. A model case in riverbank searches are the "Green River Murder Investigations," a series of homicides attributed to Gary Leon Ridgeway, carried out in the state of Washington, United States. See WD Haglund, DG Reichert and DT Reay, 1990, Recovery of decomposed and skeletal human remains in the "Green River Murder" Investigation: Implications for medical examiner/coroner and police, *American Journal of Forensic Medical Pathology, 11*(1), pp. 35–43. Also see WD Haglund, TD Reay, and CC Snow,1987, Identification of Serial Homicide Victims in the "Green River Murder" Investigation, *Journal of Forensic Sciences, 32*(6), pp. 1666–1675.

15. The definition of mass grave used by the authors of this article is provided by S. Schmitt: "A mass grave can be defined as one that contains the remains of more than one victim who share some trait connected with the cause and manner of death." (2002:279).

of one mass gravesite in the country do not always correspond to one mass disappearance. While there are instances of group disappearances followed by collective burials in one gravesite, there are many examples of individuals being buried at one particular gravesite that is not related to the same incident. Increasingly in Colombia, people are individually and systematically killed from different places in one general region, and are buried in specific areas allocated by responsible parties. As the years go by and cases accumulate, these burial sites gradually become clandestine cemeteries, holding the remains of dozens, if not hundreds, of disappeared individuals. Thus, seemingly discrete and unconnected episodes of individual disappearances are related by the acts of perpetrators who bury these individuals in specific sites. Such clandestine cemeteries, which may contain many individual or mass graves, are often located in specific areas of armed control, such as *haciendas* (a large estate, often for livestock or agricultural plantations) or encampments (Fig. 8-3 and 8-4).

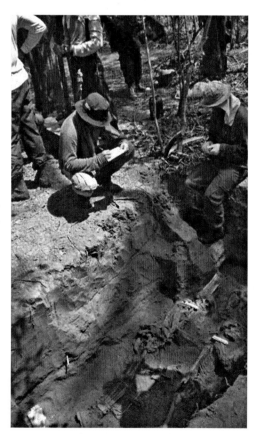

Figure 8-3. Gravesite found within a *hacienda* located in northwestern Colombia. Credit: EQUITAS.

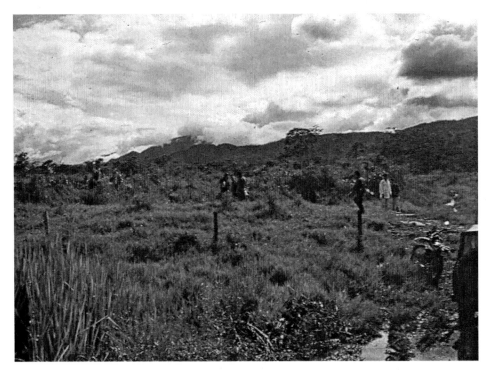

Figure 8-4. Archaeological survey carried out to locate mass graves in eastern Colombia. Credit: Andrés Patiño Umaña.

Clandestine cemeteries in these areas are sometimes concealed by perpetrators through modifications to the landscape, such as agricultural crops, artificial lakes, or wild vegetation coverage caused by abandonment (Figs. 8-5 and 8-6).

This burial pattern has become increasingly public during the last couple of years, and has recently garnered the attention of the United Nations.[16]

---

16. The 2005 UN Report of the High Commissioner for Human Rights on the Situation of Human Rights in Colombia states that allegations of forced disappearances became "more evident a certain time after the events, through the discovery of clandestine graves, individual or collective, such as those of Salazar, Sardinata, and in the rural area of Cúcuta (Norte de Santander) and in San Onofre (Sucre)." See E/CN.4/2006/9, January 20, 2006, Annex III, paragraph 31.

See also the UN Working Group on Enforced and Involuntary Disappearances' 2006 report on its mission to Colombia: "Reportedly, thousands of graveyards containing bodies of missing and disappeared persons still exist all over the country. Apparently, information gleaned from the general public about such graves reveals a more widespread pattern than previously known." UNWGEID 2006, IV D, Paragraph 51.

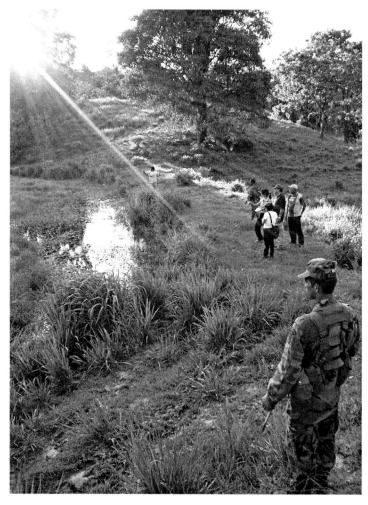

Figure 8-5. Archaeological survey carried out in a *hacienda* located in central Colombia, in an area where an artificial lake had been created. Credit: EQUITAS.

During 2004 and 2005, there were several discoveries of clandestine cemeteries located throughout rural areas of Colombia,[17] particularly

17. This does not mean that this burial pattern is exclusive to the Colombian countryside. In 2003, mass graves created by paramilitaries were found in the *Comuna 13*, a slum area in the outskirts of the city of Medellín, province of Antioquia. For more information, see "La maquinaria de las desapariciones en la Comuna 13 y las fosas." *El Colombiano* [Regional newspaper – Medellín], August 13, 2003. This case was also documented in the 2003 UN Report of the High Commissioner for Human Rights on the Situation of Human Rights in Colombia, E/CN.4/2004/13, February 17, 2004.

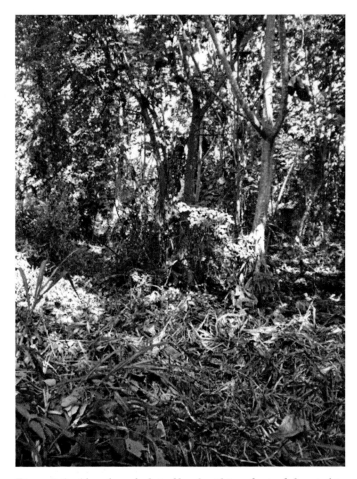

Figure 8-6. Abandoned plot of land within a *hacienda* located in northwestern Colombia, where wild vegetation has covered a gravesite. Credit: EQUITAS.

in areas of paramilitary and guerrilla control.[18] Perhaps the most publicized example is located in San Onofre, in the province of Sucre, where

---

18. Clandestine cemeteries are not, however, a recent phenomenon. Colombian non-governmental organizations report that this burial pattern in paramilitary-owned *haciendas* may date back to the mid and late-1980s, particularly in the town of Puerto López, province of Meta. See *Colombia Nunca Más*, 2000. Tomo I, Zona 7. Colombian guerrilla groups use similar methods, and have done so for an equally long time. A clear example are the mass graves found in the town of Tacueyo, province of Cauca, where the command of the Ricardo Franco guerrilla front assassinated hundreds of its members and indigenous civilians in the mid-1980s and buried these individuals in a clandestine cemetery. See "Colombia says it found more mass graves," *The New York Times*, December 18, 1985.

a clandestine gravesite discovered in 2005 at the Hacienda El Palmar is believed to hold the remains of hundreds of individuals disappeared since 1998.[19] Some of the remains found in San Onofre were disarticulated through dismemberment, and were deposited in small, shallow graves.[20] Other recent findings, such as in El Tarra, in the province of Norte de Santander, confirm that there are hundreds of disappeared individuals buried in specific areas of the country exposed to years of continuous violence, and controlled by Colombian armed factions.[21] Several mass graves have been discovered in banana and African palm plantations in Ciénaga, province of Magdalena; the authorities do not rule out the possibility of finding yet more graves in this area.[22] At the time of writing, Colombian authorities have found a large clandestine cemetery in the township of La Gabarra, department of Norte de Santander.[23]

The formation of these clandestine cemeteries is becoming a hallmark of the Colombian context. These aforementioned examples are not unique, unrelated incidents; they are illustrative of a regional trend regularly used by armed factions.

---

19. For more information, please refer to the article by Juan Forero "Colombia unearthing plight of its disappeared," *The New York Times*, August 10, 2005. Also see "La hacienda El Palmar, en San Onofre (Sucre), está sembrada de historias del terror paramilitar," *El Tiempo* [Colombian national newspaper], April 17, 2005.

20. The 2006 UN Report of the High Commissioner for Human Rights on the Situation of Human Rights in Colombia stated that, in San Onofre, "a significant number of corpses were found in graves containing one or two bodies, buried less than one meter below ground and which had been dismembered. A number of bodies showed signs of torture. Among these were recent victims who seemed to have been killed less than a year ago. This demonstrates the persistence of this practice, which is generally under-recorded." See E/CN.4/2006/009, Annex III, paragraph 23.

21. For more information, please refer to "Cerca de 300 cuerpos están enterrados en más de 40 fosas comunes en las veredas de El Tarra," *El Tiempo* [Colombian national newspaper], November 5, 2004.

22. For more information, please refer to "Mass graves unearthed in Colombia," BBC News, February 15, 2006 and "Los restos oseos de 20 personas fueron encontrados en diferentes fosas comunes en Tucurinca," *El Tiempo* [Colombian national newspaper], February 12, 2006.

23. For more information, please refer to "Colombian investigators find mass grave," *The Associated Press*, April 11, 2006. Also see "En 14 fosas comunes se han encontrado ya los cadáveres de 179 personas asesinadas," *El Tiempo* [Colombian national newspaper], April 12, 2006.and "Exhumaciones de Fiscalía en Catatumbo animaron a familias a desenterrar sus muertos de fosas comunes," *El Tiempo* [Colombian national newspaper], April 15, 2006.

CURRENT PROBLEMS IN OFFICIAL RESPONSES TO FINDING DISAPPEARED INDIVIDUALS

Given the country's conflictive environment, it is little wonder that Colombia poses one of the most difficult contexts for searching and recovering human remains when compared with other situations globally. Aside from the challenges described above, ongoing violence in Colombian rural areas poses logistical difficulties for judicial investigators, who often have to work in active conflict zones and under the pressure of armed groups. Landmines are scattered in many of Colombia's conflict regions,[24] sometimes overlapping with areas where mass gravesites may be found. Colombia's diverse geographic landscape, which ranges from plains and mountainous areas to deserts and tropical forests, also sets complicated settings for archaeological fieldwork (Fig. 8-7).

Despite having judicial investigators that for the most part are well-trained and technically qualified, Colombian governmental offices fall short in responding to the sheer number of disappearance cases that require forensic archaeologists or anthropologists. This can be explained in part by the lack of material resources, logistical capacity, facilities, equipment and available personnel. However, Colombian authorities also lack effective plans of action required to properly address the challenges of finding disappeared individuals. This is evident in the lack of coordination between governmental offices dedicated to investigate disappearances in Colombia, which may lead to competing and overlapping activities.[25] Forensic specialists working inside Colombia's judicial system, public offices and police forces often do not share information or collaborate in search and recovery efforts on the ground. All these circumstances lead to improvisation, mishandling and other negligent shortcomings in forensic investigations.

---

24. Colombia is one of the countries most heavily-affected by landmines worldwide. According to the Landmine Monitor Report 2005 from the International Campaign to Ban Landmines, Colombia is the third country after Afghanistan and Cambodia with the greatest number of landmine casualties. This report is available at www.icbl.org/lm/

25. In its report about its mission to Colombia, the UN Working Group on Enforced and Involuntary Disappearances identified that, for the proper implementation of legislation regarding disappearances, "the problems include: having too many institutions and agencies operating within and across different arms of government, including the legislative, executive and judicial, each with their own competing programmes and missions; inadequate staffing; inadequate funding; lack of central coordination; poor inter-agency communication; fragmentation of authority, with heads of the various agencies viewing them as their own power bases." See UNWGEID 2006, IV, B, paragraph 43.

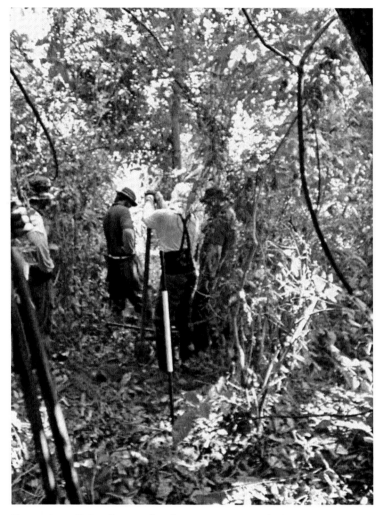

Figure 8-7. Colombian judicial investigators probing gravesite areas in the same location (see Figure 8-6). Credit: EQUITAS.

Although Colombian legislation provides some tools for the creation of proper search strategies for missing individuals,[26] there are several

___

26. One such example is the National Search Commission for the Search of Disappeared Individuals was a result of Law 589 of 2000, which formally criminalized the disappearance of individuals, genocide, and forced displacement in Colombia. Aside from the judicial institutions mentioned above, the Commission also includes public entities such as the Public Ombudsman's Office, the Inspector General's Office, the Office of the Vice-President for Human Rights, the Office of the President for Personal Freedom, the Ministry of Defense, and two non-governmental organizations, the Association of Relatives of the Detained and Disappeared (ASFADDES) and the Colombian Commission of Jurists.

problems evident in the implementation of these laws. Perhaps the main one is not having a complete and comprehensive register of who is missing in Colombia. There are currently several separate databases on disappearances being maintained by governmental agencies. The National Institute of Legal Medicine and Forensic Sciences currently houses a register of disappeared individuals and unidentified corpses, which lists ". . . identity of the disappeared persons, the date and time of the disappearance, as well as lists of corpses, unburied human remains and unidentified persons, with an indication of the date of the findings and other relevant data." (UNWGEID, 2006, Paragraph 34). However, the National Institute's register is partial and deficient. This is partly attributable to Colombia's conflict situation, where the presence of armed groups makes information-gathering on behalf of Colombian government authorities and the production of case statements from affected relatives difficult. But under-registration is largely due to internal problems in state entities, where records are often incomplete and outdated. There are also strong deficiencies in information-crossing between and within Colombian governmental offices. Legislation for the creation of a national registry of disappeared individuals in Colombia (known as the *Registro Único de Personas Desaparecidas*[27]) was approved in 2005. While such a registry is beneficial, its full potential cannot be appraised until this legislation is implemented.

Until this registry exists, this lack of comprehensive knowledge will continue to cause problems in the investigation of disappeared individuals for Colombian authorities, particularly when confronting a clandestine cemetery. The absence of a complete picture regarding who is missing has direct implications for the application of forensic archaeology and anthropology in the recovery and identification of disappeared individuals, as described below.

However, before describing these problems, it is worth drawing attention to the ongoing debate with reference to the objectives of forensic archaeology and anthropology (as well as other forensic sciences) when investigating disappearances. On the one hand, forensic scientists are called in to collect human remains at a mass grave to personally identify missing persons; on the other, human remains are treated as contextual evidence to be used in a court of law in the prosecution of perpetrators (Doretti and Snow, 2003). This humanitarian/legal differentiation is

---

27. See *Reglamentación del artículo 9 de la Ley 589 del 2000, Decreto Número 4218 de 2005.*

largely set by international tribunals and truth commissions that hire forensic scientists to produce evidence for criminal investigations carried out in these legal settings, where identification is not a priority (Haglund, 2002:258). There have been archaeologists who support this differentiation, understanding the former as an "exhumation" and the latter as an "excavation" (Juhl, 2005), and even favoring the production of forensic evidence over the humanitarian need of identifying missing individuals (Dirkmaat et al., 2005). In Colombia, however, such legal and humanitarian goals are not mutually exclusive, but rather are dependant of each other, as this chapter intends to illustrate.

PROBLEMS IN RECOVERY OF MATERIALS AND IDENTIFICATION OF REMAINS FROM CLANDESTINE CEMETERIES

Not knowing which individuals are missing leads to partial archaeological recovery – and potential loss – of remains and material evidence found *in situ* at clandestine cemeteries in Colombia. Colombian judicial institutions, implementing strictly traditional manual archaeological methods (Fig. 8-8), have demonstrated logistical capacity and technical ability in planning large-scale excavations, evident not only in cases like San Onofre, but also previously in landmark cases such as Bojayá and the Palace of Justice.[28] Yet regretfully, in some cases, Colombian judicial investigators may temporarily suspend or terminate excavations without a complete recovery of all remains at a particular site.[29]

---

28. The Bojayá case refers to the May 2002 FARC pipe-bomb attack in the small hamlet of Bojayá, province of Chocó, where 119 people were killed inside a church, most of whom were women and children. For more information, see BBC News, "Fear grows for Colombian civilians," May 6, 2002.

The Palace of Justice case refers to the 1985 siege of Colombia's Supreme Court and the two-day military counterattack, where hostage magistrates, guerrilla members, and dozens of innocent civilians were killed or disappeared. Both cases required large-scale forensic interventions – the 1998 Palace of Justice exhumation in Bogotá's *Cementerio del Sur*, where victims' remains were allegedly buried, was at its time the largest forensic excavation undertaken by Colombian judicial investigators. For more information, see the 1998 Annual Report of Argentine Forensic Anthropology Team (EAAF), particularly pages 20-23. Available at www.eaaf.org.

29. At the time of this writing, a congressional representative was calling the Colombian government to question for suspending the investigation at San Onofre. See "El Palmar, campo de exterminio en Sucre." *El Espectador* [Colombian national newspaper], February 12, 2006.

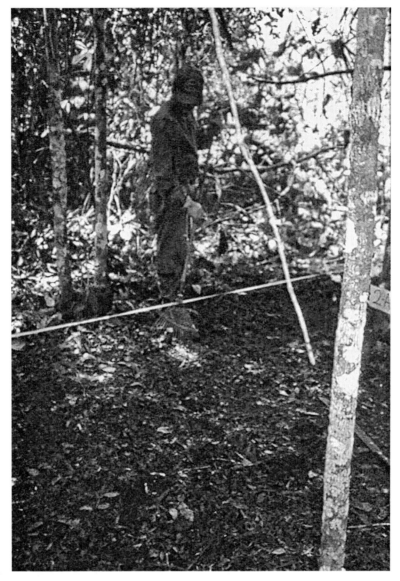

Figure 8-8. Colombian judicial official clearing surface foliage from excavation site. Credit: Andrés Patiño Umaña.

The same investigators may also carry out individual spot searches for
missing persons, favoring a case-by-case recovery rather than a complete excavation – even when the presence of a clandestine cemetery in
that location is evident. Both situations inevitably lead to the loss of
valuable information of not only the buried remains and evidence, but

also of interment and site formation processes (Spennemann and Franke, 1995). Given that an archaeological intervention is by definition destructive (Hunter, 1997), clandestine cemeteries require the utmost care in the application of archaeological techniques for the recovery of remains and evidence (Skinner, 1987) and normative guidelines for appropriate site management (Skinner et al., 2003).

Carrying out a partial investigation brings with it the cost of unrecoverable site destruction without the benefit of complete remains recovery. However, partial investigation can also lead to the destruction of evidence by third parties. In a conflict situation like Colombia, where armed factions are still present in the very areas in which disappearances are committed, forensic missions often attract the unwanted attention of perpetrators. This increases the vulnerability of a crime site, as perpetrators may subsequently remove or destroy the evidence of crimes they have committed.

Not knowing who is missing also leads to the impossibility of identification, as well as to the potential loss of remains and evidence. Many large-scale excavations are also regrettably unsuccessful with reference to affecting the identifications of all the victims involved, because of a lack of information as to who is missing. Identification is the Achilles' heel of these investigations, where human remains may be recovered but not successfully identified. Colombian governmental officials are left with no choice but to temporarily store remains at relevant institutions, and later bury them in less than appropriate locations – such as in a mass grave at the back of a cemetery.

NNs in Colombian Cemeteries: The Unfortunate Cost of Not Knowing Who Is Missing

Individuals that are not identified by Colombian authorities, and are left unclaimed are regularly buried in the back of Colombian public cemeteries as "NNs" (an acronym which stands for "no name");[30] the system in turn does not have the capacity to store large amounts of remains in official installations for long periods of time. Such unidentified deaths are not only a result of Colombia's conflict, but also of other criminal homicides, emergencies or natural disasters. Hundreds, if not thousands

---

30. The NN burial phenomenon is common in other areas of Latin America, such as Argentina, as documented in C Snow and M Bihurriet 1992.

of "NNs," are buried in Colombian cemeteries every year (see Chapter 9 of this volume for studies and results obtained on NNs in Argentina).

While current legislation in some areas of Colombia now requires cemeteries to bury non-identified individuals in separate graves,[31] most are still buried in a manner throughout the country that does not always comply with international recommendations.[32] Thus, the remains of disappeared individuals are often found commingled with other remains in collective mass graves located in Colombian cemeteries, where the individuality of the remains may not always be adequately preserved and indicated. Poor cemetery records also make it extremely difficult to track when and where remains were buried (Fig. 8-9). Morgue files and judicial institutions tend to not be much more reliable in providing information. As mentioned earlier, remains may be found, but are then poorly analyzed by Colombian judicial investigators. This leads to the virtual documentary "disappearance" of these people, as well as to the loss of their remains – and evidence of the killings and other associated crimes committed against these disappeared individuals (Snow and Bihurriet, 1992).

The costs of this careless burial behavior in cemeteries are enormous for investigative purposes. A tragic example is the Pueblo Bello case. Pueblo Bello is a town from which 43 *campesinos* (peasants) disappeared in 1990 by a paramilitary group led by Fidel Castaño Gil. The *campesinos* were allegedly tortured and assassinated in Fidel Castaño's hacienda, known as *Las Tangas*, located in the outskirts of the city of Montería, in the province of Córdoba. In April 1990, Colombian police carried out an exhumation in *Las Tangas*, where the remains of 24 men were allegedly recovered – using a bulldozer. Six were identified by visual recognition, and the remaining eighteen, all badly destroyed due to the effects of heavy machinery, were subsequently buried as NNs in a cemetery in Montería.

Since then, four government-led investigations related to the Pueblo Bello case at the Montería cemetery have been enacted, all of which have been unsuccessful in finding and recovering remains linked to this case. In all of these investigations, judicial authorities sifted through a mass grave containing hundreds of buried individuals – of which there

---

31. In the case of cemetery regulations for Bogotá, see *Reglamentación de cementerios y funerarias, Decreto No. 391,* July 3, 1991.

32. See *Management of Dead Bodies in Disaster Situations* (Disaster Manuals and Guideline Series No. 5). Washington, DC: Pan-American Health Organization and World Health Organization, 2004, pp. 129–181.

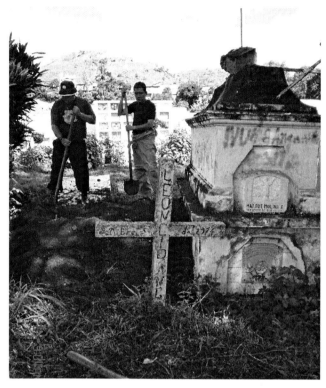

Figure 8-9. Exhumation carried out in the "NN" area of a public cemetery in northeastern Colombia. Credit: EQUITAS.

were no records retained by the cemetery administration. The Inter-American Court of Human Rights has recently issued a ruling for the Pueblo Bello case, in which it found against the Colombian government, and identified judicial authorities as negligent, not only in the obviously poor recovery of remains *in situ* in *Las Tangas*, but also in the subsequent handling of the bodies taken to Montería.[33]

The Pueblo Bello case is representative of the fate of many of Colombian nationals. Their remains may be recovered, only to be lost again within a mass grave located at a public cemetery. When particular cases advance years after the events transpired, Colombian judicial investigators often struggle to find the remains of missing people in the midst of cemeteries throughout the country, a task demanding in time, per-

---

33. Corte Interamericana de Derechos Humanos. Sentencia *Caso de la Masacre Pueblo Bello vs. Colombia,* January 31, 2006, paragraphs 173–178.

sonnel, and economic resources. Thus, although the remains of missing individuals may be found by Colombian authorities, they will continue to be disappeared as unidentified NN's.[34]

It is clear that not knowing who is missing in Colombia contributes to a lack of success in investigations carried out at clandestine cemeteries to recover disappeared individuals. This lack of success manifests itself in two ways: (1) the recovery of evidence and materials as legal evidence, and (2) the identification of individuals for humanitarian purposes. On the one hand, not knowing who is missing leads to mechanical excavations at a clandestine cemetery without a quantitative yardstick from which to measure the complete recovery of remains and materials. Evidence and remains can thus be lost, both through archaeological destruction and by third parties. On the other hand, not knowing who is missing denies the possibility of identification, leading also to the loss of remains and evidence in the confines of a public cemetery. It is this vicious cycle that leads many official investigations of disappeared individuals to fail.

SCIENTIFIC CONTRIBUTIONS TO COLOMBIAN DISAPPERANCE CASES

When confronting a clandestine cemetery, knowing who is missing helps to answer the two main questions necessary for recovery and identification efforts. These are: (1) who of Colombia's missing may be buried at this site, and (2) what is the complete picture of what needs to be recovered. In addition to this, application of forensic archaeology and anthropology, in conjunction with the use of other scientific disciplines, can help remedy – and avoid – the problems in recovery and identification that characterize official investigations of clandestine cemeteries in Colombia.

Determining Who is Missing

There are two sources of information on the missing in Colombia:

---

34. In its report about its mission to Colombia, the UN Working Group on Enforced and Involuntary Disappearances stated that, "a number of disappeared persons might have been among the many bodies which had been found [by Colombian authorities] and never identified." See UNWGEID 2006, IV D, Paragraph 51.

general reports on missing persons, and the antemortem data of these individuals. General reports on missing individuals, preferably those from regions around clandestine graves, should be collected in order to determine an estimated figure of the number of disappeared individuals. Such documentation can come from a variety of sources, such as records from morgues, hospitals, and judicial institutions,[35] reports from human rights and civil society organizations, and direct testimonies from families involved.

After getting a grasp of how many individuals may be missing at one particular site, plans for antemortem data collection may then fall into place. The names of some missing individuals will be provided by the reports used to calculate the "universe" of missing individuals, yet there may also be others who need to be found. Antemortem data of both named and unnamed individuals will need to be collected in as many cases as possible, through the use of social networks, such as government offices, churches, and civil society organizations. These records on the missing and their antemortem information need to be as complete as possible on the outset of an investigation, be it at a local, regional or national level,[36] in order to improve the chances of identifying remains that are recovered.

Scientific Prospects and Limitations of Recovering and Identifying Individuals

In their article "Exhumation of mass graves: Balancing legal and humanitarian needs," Stover and Shigekane (2004:88) state that, ". . . [International forensic teams] brought with them new technologies and scientific advances designed to bring greater accuracy to their investigations. Satellite imagery made it possible to generate maps to be used in pinpointing graves hidden in remote locations. Electronic mapping systems had replaced the archaeological technique of a baseline and string grid, which meant the teams could now save time and produce more

---

35. M Doretti, M. and I Cano, 1995. Violations of the right to life in Haiti, 1985–1995. Unpublished paper presented to the Haitian National Commission for Truth and Justice, as cited in Ball 1996.

36. The elaboration of complete, centralized databases of disappeared individuals is recommended by the International Committee of the Red Cross. See ICRC, *The Missing: Action to resolve the problem of people unaccounted for as a result of armed conflict or internal violence and to assist their families.* ICRC/The Missing/ 12.2002/EN/6. Available at www.icrc.org/eng

accurate data . . . advancements in DNA analysis meant that scientists could identify some remains that had confounded more traditional anthropological methods."

The promises of such scientific advances in the investigation of mass graves serve to shed light on the Colombian situation. Recovering and identifying remains in Colombia poses many challenges, and positive results may not always be achievable. Difficult archaeological contexts frequently make recoveries a complex task, and the lack of antemortem data may make positive identifications unattainable in many cases. Regardless of such issues, scientific disciplines mentioned by Stover and Shigekane (2004), such as satellite imagery and genetics, in addition to other fields such as statistics, may prove useful in complementing such forensic investigations, so as to minimize the possibility of failure.

The Use of Remote-sensing Information

Large-scale excavations can be better planned, often with concrete information pertaining to the location and size of mass graves. This is particularly true in Colombia, where a clandestine cemetery can cover a considerable area of land and hold a number of individual or collective gravesites. New archaeological data acquisition techniques, such as aerial photography and remote sensing, can also be used for planning excavations at a distance. Analyzing images obtained by aircraft and satellite observation can assist in the determination of exact locations, in addition to areas of disturbance in ground surface composition, thereby adding information to known sites difficult to discover at ground-level. This allows investigators to design an archaeological plan of action prior to going to the area in question.

Aerial photography and satellite imagery complement the application of traditional archaeological techniques in finding of remains and contextual evidence, particularly in burial depositional contexts. It is not within the scope of this chapter to carry out a comprehensive review of applicable archaeological techniques (Owsley, 1995; Dirkmaat and Adovasio, 1997), particularly in reference to the excavation of mass gravesites (Haglund, 2002; Haglund et al., 2001; Hunter and Cox, 2005; Schmitt, 2002; Skinner, 1987), which have been excellently discussed elsewhere. Colombian mass gravesites require the proper application of archaeological methods, as well as the careful documentation and analysis of stratigraphy and the spatial distribution of remains and contextual evidence, in order to guarantee a rigorous recovery of the gravesite's contents and a complete understanding of the temporal sequence of their deposit and the site's formation.[37] However, these can prove to be difficult to implement in Colombian conflict regions, where the attention of armed factions in such areas should not be unnecessarily drawn. Thus, instead of determining the area to be investigated in the field, forensic missions should attempt to plan the excavation as much as possible prior to commencing work.

Remote sensing has been used in traditional archaeological investigations (Banning, 2002), as well as in the detection of human remains (Davenport, 2001; Killam, 2004). They have also been applied to locate graves in post-conflict regions worldwide. Satellite imagery and spectral analysis have been used in Bosnia-Herzegovina to identify patterns of soil disturbances indicative of the location of mass graves resulting from conflict in the former Yugoslavia.[38] In Colombia's active conflict, aerial photography and remote sensing may prove to be an excellent non-invasive method for planning excavations without going to the ground and alerting armed actors of attempts to find graves, reducing the possibility for evidence destruction. Chronological series of satellite images can also be matched with information on temporal and spatial trends found in statistical analyses of disappearance records. Yet because searches in Colombia take place in varied environments, as described earlier, these methods will probably prove to be most useful in large expanses of land not used for intensive agriculture. More testing is required to assure that such methods will be successful in Colombia, but the potential benefits in responding to specific challenges due to the country's conflict should not be overlooked.

The Use of Genetic Testing

In many areas of the world where violent conflict has left behind

---

37. As stated by Dirkmaat and Adovasio 1997, the archaeological principles applicable to outdoor excavation sites are: (1) the delineation of the site's stratigraphy from observed stratification, (2) the maintenance of context, and (3) the establishment of any associations between recovered materials. These same principles are highlighted as relevant to mass grave excavations in Dirkmaat et al., 2005.
38. For more information, please refer to "Experts investigate new methods of using satellite images to locate mass grave sites," *The Associated Press*, May 31, 2005 and "New way to find mass graves in Bosnia," *The Associated Press*, August 17, 2005. See also International Commission on Missing Persons, "ICMP finds improved methods for locating mass graves," Press release, August 16, 2005. Available at www.ic-mp.org

scores of missing individuals, positive identification of all victims may not always be possible (Haglund, 2002:258). Given the scarcity of antemortem data in rural Colombian populations, such as dental and medical records, positive identification is not always possible through anthropological methods. DNA analysis is thus the best way to identify bodies, and has been regularly used in human rights investigations worldwide (Boles et al., 1995; Harvey and King, 2002; Primorac et al., 1996). Yet, given the high costs of genetic testing in Colombia, presumptive identification is often more feasible than positive identification through DNA.

Despite this situation, positive identification should be a goal of forensic investigations of disappeared individuals. Large-scale genetic testing is costly, but not impossible. New genetic testing techniques used in countries where antemortem information on large numbers of disappeared individuals is partial, such as Bosnia-Herzegovina (Huffine et al., 2001), allow for mass identifications of victims to be made without the use of individual DNA records, making large-scale genetic testing feasible. Kinship analyses substitute the needs of previous technologies, where group testing was not possible, and where genetic samples from immediate relatives were required to identify an individual (Leclair, 2004). It is worth emphasizing that DNA analysis forces the Colombian authorities to carry out rigorous and accurate documentation, recovery, storage, and maintenance of remains, both for necessary anthropological analyses, as well as to ensure the viability of future inquiries using DNA technology.

The Use of Statistics

In order for DNA analysis to be remotely successful, forensic scientists need to have an idea of who the remains found at a mass gravesite belong to. Genetics, as well as any form of forensic identification, is based on a one-to-one correspondence between found remains and the biological information of who those remains may belong to. Thus, aside from knowing who is missing, it is necessary to correlate these records with specific gravesites, in order to potentially match the profiles of the missing with remains found. To do this, statistics can be a useful tool in Colombia, as has proven to be the case in other places, such as Argentina (Joyce and Stover, 1991; Snow and Bihurriet, 1992).

Statistical analysis is useful in forensic investigations of disappeared individuals for two reasons. The first is that, through a complete register of missing persons and mass gravesites in Colombia, these fields can identify temporal and spatial trends in order to match missing individuals with particular dates and sites. In other words, quantitative analysis can establish time-space trends of missing person data (i.e., where and when these disappearances took place) that can be matched with the date formation and location of mass gravesites. This can allow investigators to establish hypotheses about the identity of persons found in certain burials.

The second reason statistics are useful in such forensic investigations is to determine under-registration. In a country such as Colombia, where there is a significant level of underreporting, statistical analysis provides a necessary framework, and facilitates understanding of the dimension of the problem at a regional level, based on limited records. The number of cases of particular human rights violations in a given time and place can be elucidated through the use of incomplete or distorted data (Samuelson and Spirer, 1992). Thus, with only a partial base of information, statistical analysis may assist in establishing the general universe of missing persons in Colombia – and help guide information-gathering pertaining to unknown cases. Similar large-scale analyses (Ball, 1996; Ball et al., 2000) have been carried out in other areas worldwide, to determine the "universe" of certain crimes, such as conflict-related deaths.[39] These large-scale methods of analysis have been used in the contexts of truth commissions, such as in East Timor (Silva and Ball, 2006).

THE NEEDS OF FAMILIES AND COMMUNITIES IN COLOMBIAN DISAPPEARANCE CASES

The disappearance of a relative, and the lack of their remains causes unresolved grief and emotional strain for many families and communities in Colombia (MSF, 2006:34). Without the remains of their missing loved ones, victims are not only left without legal reparation for these crimes, but perhaps more seriously, without the possibility of completing closure (Stover et al., 2003). In reality "One of the most powerful

---

39. For an example of the statistical calculation of the death toll from Peru's civil war, see J Knight, 2003, "Statistical model leaves Peru counting the cost of civil war," *Nature, 425*(6953), p. 6.

barriers to healing, or reconciliation, and rebuilding of societies following [war or civil unrest] is the psychologically unsettling issue of missing persons. Families of the disappeared are suspended in a "no-man's-land" of psychological and spiritual existence. This is compounded by a perceived lack of justice, as none has been administered to those responsible for the disappearance (and hence unknown status) of their loved one(s)" (Keough et al., 2004:271).

Some families of missing individuals continue to live in the same areas where their relative(s) disappeared, and where the perpetrators may still be active. Such families also endure the stress of living in a conflict zone, vulnerable to threats and the fear of reprisals from armed factions if they attempt to search for their loved ones. Mental health constitutes a grave public health problem, particularly in conflict areas of Colombia, where violence is the leading cause of death. International mental health experts have reported that considerable numbers of individuals inhabiting these violence-stricken areas seek medical assistance for physical symptoms often experienced by those forced to live in fear (Reilley and Morote, 2004:2577). Many of these individuals rarely get general medical assistance, much less psychological support. Thus, families and communities in Colombia often face the double burden of grieving the loss of a missing loved one, as well as struggling for day-to-day survival amidst the violence. Victims are left without a feeling of control, not only because of the environment of terror in which they live, but also because they lack the support of an agency which actively searches for their loved one(s).

Recovering remains is a key element of assisting families of the disappeared to gain control over what has happened (Beristain,1999:111), an event that will have a multiplier effect throughout the community. Although disappearances in Colombia occur in a systematic individual manner, the regional manifestation of disappearance and effects on many populations throughout the country make disappearances a collective experience (Summerfield, 1995) with an impact on a community's "social fabric" (Beristain,1999). The very regional manifestation of disappearances, and the formation of clandestine graves in Colombia require community-based participation in forensic investigations. Burying remains and carrying out memorials can also prove to be essential in restoring the community's physical and social environment (Pollack, 2003). Thus, communities undergoing search and exhumation processes require special support from psychosocial experts (Keough and Samuels,

2004),[40] a process which has been monitored by local and international organizations.[41]

Family and community participation has increasingly been identified by forensic experts to be a vital part for investigatory success in conflict settings (Stover and Shigekane, 2002; 2004; Stover et al., 2003). In Colombia, participation of families is fundamental to forensic investigations. On the one hand, identification is not possible without ante-mortem information of a victim's family, or, by default, a genetic sample. On the other hand, remains need to be identified and returned to families, so that they can properly grieve the loss of a loved one. The participation of families needs to be facilitated by scientific investigations that promote the use of procedures respectful to the needs of family members, where relatives are active participants in all stages of the investigation, from the collection of antemortem data and identification (Keough et al., 2000) to the burial of remains (Pollack, 2003). Here, as in other places, timely collaborative proposals to meet the humanitarian needs of families and the legal needs of forensic investigators will need to be implemented (Keough et al., 2004). In summation, it is essential for families to participate in the search process,[42] and to be "actively involved in the consultative and decision-making processes of locating, exhuming, reburying, and memorializing their dead" (Stover and Shigekane, 2004:98).

Complete recovery and identification of remains also fulfills the rights of victims in knowing what has happened. Reconstruction of the events from material found in mass graves that relates to the disappearance of their missing loved ones is not only legally relevant, but also historically relevant (Juhl, 2005:22). The right of families to know the fate of their

---

40. This need has led to the formation of several groups in countries plagued by conflict-related disappearances, such as the *Equipo Comunitario para la Acción Participativa* (ECAP) in Guatemala and the Amani Trust in Zimbabwe, which aim to support communities undergoing exhumation and/or the search for their missing loved ones.

41. See "Monitoring of the community and psychosocial impact of exhumation processes of mass graves in Latin America: An international collaborative project based on local NGOs work." Paper presented in 2005 to the Psychosocial Working Group by the Community Action Group (GAC) – Spain; Community Studies and Psychosocial Action Team (ECAP) – Guatemala; Solomon Asch Center for the Study of Ethnopolitical Conflict – USA; and Child Mental Health Care Program (PASMI) – Peru. Available at www.forcedmigration.org/psychosocial/PWGinfo.htm

42. See V Nesiah, 2002, *The Missing: Overcoming the tensions between family needs and judicial procedures*, ICRC/The Missing/09.2002/EN/8. Also refer to ICRC, *The Missing: Action to resolve the problem of people unaccounted for as a result of armed conflict or internal violence and to assist their families*. ICRC/The Missing/ 12.2002/EN/6. Available at www.icrc.org/eng

relatives also includes knowing completely what happened and to whom (Fondebrider and Doretti, 2001), and for which complete recovery and identification becomes necessary.

CONCLUSION

The unfortunate result of many current investigations regarding the disappeared in Colombia is that costly and time-consuming forensic missions are unfruitful, valuable information is lost, and additional anguish is created to the families of victims who must already bear the absence of a loved one. This chapter hopes to establish that investigations of disappeared individuals in Colombia will only be effective when knowing who is missing is a part of the strategy. In order for the application of forensic archaeology and anthropology in investigations of clandestine cemeteries to be successful, both in recovering evidence and identifying remains, it is necessary to have information on who is missing, in order to know what to recover as legal evidence and how to identify what is found, thereby fulfilling the humanitarian needs of families. Not having this information implies the possible loss of remains and evidence *in situ*, or its subsequent loss in a public cemetery through NN burials.

Recovering and identifying the remains of all missing individuals in Colombia is not only daunting, but perhaps impossible. Despite this, no tasks with regards to the proper collection and identification of remains should be sacrificed. As stated by Dirkmaat et al., "The perception is that if a detailed forensic archaeological recovery of such features is attempted, the sheer size of the feature, the large number of victims interred, and apparent complexity of the feature will result in tremendous overruns in both time and resources . . . [which] is often couched in terms of delaying the return of victims to families," (2005:15). However, knowing who is missing, along with adequate planning "with a scientific/forensic perspective" of Colombian clandestine cemeteries should ultimately lead to the acquisition of "proper, contextually-based recovery of forensically significant evidence" that should allow, if not enhance, the possibility of remains identification (Dirkmaat et al., 2005:15). In other words, the appropriate forensic investigations of the disappeared in Colombia "should encompass all those observations and procedures which are necessary and practicable to enable . . . identification of the human remains," a task which in no way "derogates from the serious justice-related purposes" of these investigations (Cordner and McKelvie, 2002:878). Thus, legal-related purposes match the humanitarian needs of families in these investigations, and together, help to conclusively resolve the issue of missing individuals in Colombia. It is in this way that forensic investigations of disappearances transcend the legal and criminally punitive aspects of remains and material recovery, and have broader impacts for societal healing (McEvoy and Conway, 2004), an aspect of deep-seated importance in a country plagued by decades-long conflict such as Colombia.

REFERENCES

Ball, P. (1996). *Who did what to whom? Planning and implementing a large scale human rights data project.* Washington, D.C.: American Association for the Advancement of Science.

Ball, P., Spirer, H.F., and Spirer, L. (2000). *Making the case: Investigating large scale human rights violations using information systems and data analysis.* Washington, D.C.: American Association for the Advancement of Science.

Banning, E.B. (2002). *Archaeological survey: Manuals in archaeological method, theory and technique.* New York: Kluwer Academic/ Plenum Publishers.

Bassett, H.E., and Manheim, M.H. (2002). Fluvial transport of human remains in the Lower Mississippi River. *J. Forensic Sciences, 47*(4):719–24.

Beristain, C.M. (1999). *Reconstruir el tejido social: Un enfoque crítico de la ayuda humanitaria.* Barcelona: Editorial Icaria.

Boles, T.C., Snow, C.C., and Stover, E. (1995). Forensic DNA testing on skeletal remains from mass graves: A pilot project in Guatemala. *J. Forensic Sciences, 40*(3): 349–355.

Burns, K.R. (1998). Forensic anthropology and human rights issues. In *Forensic osteology: Advances in the identification of human remains,* Reichs, K.J. (Ed.). Springfield: Charles C Thomas, pp. 63–85.

Chernick, M. (2003). Colombia: Does injustice cause violence? In *What justice? Whose justice? Fighting for fairness in Latin America,* Eckstein, S.E., and Wickham-Crowley, T.P. (Eds.). Berkeley: University of California Press, pp. 185–214.

Cordner, S., and McKelvie, H. (2002). Developing standards in international forensic work to identify missing persons. *International Review of the Red Cross, 84*(848): 867–884.

Davenport, G.C. (2001). Remote sensing applications in forensic investigations. *Historical Archaeology, 35*(1):87–100.

Dirkmaat, D.C., and Adovasio, J.M. (1997). The role of archaeology in the recovery and interpretation of human remains from an outdoor forensic setting. In *Forensic taphonomy: The postmortem fate of human remains,* Haglund, W.D., and Sorg, M.H. (Eds.). Boca Ratón: CRC Press, pp. 39–64.

Dirkmaat, D.C., Cabo, L.L., Adovasio, J.M., and Rozas, V. (2005). Commingled remains and the mass grave: Considering the benefits of forensic archaeology. Paper presented at the 57th Annual Meeting of the American Academy of Forensic Sciences, New Orleans. February 21–26.

Doretti, M., and Snow, C.C. (2003). Forensic anthropology and human rights: The Argentine experience. In *Hard evidence: Case studies in forensic anthropology*, Steadman, D.W. (Ed.). Upper Saddle River: Prentice Hall, pp. 290–310.

Ferllini, R. (1999). The role of forensic anthropology in human rights issues. In *Forensic osteological analysis: A book of case studies*, Fairgrieve, S.I. (Ed.). Springfield: Charles C Thomas, pp. 287–302.

Fondebrider, L., and Doretti, M. (2001). Truth, justice, reparation and reconciliation: A long way in third world countries. In *Archaeologies of the contemporary past*, Lucas, G., and Buchli, V. (Eds.). London: Routledge, pp. 138–144.

Haglund, W.D. (2002). Recent mass graves, an introduction. In *Advances in forensic taphonomy: Method, theory, and archaeological perspectives*, Haglund, W.D., and Sorg, M.H. (Eds.). Boca Raton: CRC Press, pp. 244–261.

Haglund, W.D., Connor, M.A., and Scott, D.D. (2001). The archaeology of contemporary mass graves. *Historical Archaeology, 35*(1):57–69.

Harvey, M., and King, M.C. (2002). The use of DNA in the identification of postmortem remains. In *Advances in forensic taphonomy: Method, theory, and archaeological perspectives*, Haglund, W.D., and Sorg, M.H. (Eds.). Boca Raton: CRC Press, pp. 474–486.

Hoshower, L.M. (1998). Forensic archaeology and the need for flexible excavation strategies: A case study. *J. Forensic Sciences, 43*(1): 53–56.

Huffine, E., Crews, J., Kennedy, B., Bomberger, K., and Zinbo, A. (2001). Mass identification of persons missing from the break-up of the Former Yugoslavia: Structure, function, and the role of the International Commission on Missing Persons. *Croatian Medical Journal, 42*:271–275.

Hunter, J. (1997). Background to forensic archaeology. In *Studies in crime: An introduction to forensic archaeology*, Hunter, J., Roberts, C., and Martin, A. (Eds.). London: BT Batsford, pp. 7–23.

Hunter, J., and Cox, M. (2005). The archaeology of mass graves. In *Forensic archaeology: Advances in theory and practice*, Hunter, J., and Cox, M. (Eds.). New York: Routledge, pp. 137–158.

ICRC (International Committee of the Red Cross) (2005). *Colombia annual report for 2004*. http://www.icrc.org.

Joyce, C., and Stover, E. (1991). *Witnesses from the grave: The stories bones tell*. Boston: Little, Brown, and Co.

Juhl, K. (2005). *The contribution of (forensic) archaeologists to human rights investigations of mass graves*. Stavanger: Museum of Archaeology. http://www.ark.museum.no/AmS-NETT/Mass_Graves2.pdf.

Keough, M., Kahn, S., and Andrejevic, A. (2000). Disclosing the truth: Informed participation in the antemortem database project for survivors of Srebrenica. *Health and Human Right, 5*(1):68–87.

Keough, M., and Samuels, M. (2004). The Kosovo family support project: Offering psychosocial support for families with missing persons. *Social Work, 49*(4):587–594.

Keough, M., Simmons, T., and Samuels, M. (2004). Missing persons in post-conflict settings: best practices for integrating psychosocial and scientific approaches. *Journal of the Royal Society for the Promotion of Health, 124*(6):271–275.

Killam, E.W. (2004). *The detection of human remains.* Springfield: Charles C Thomas.

Leclair, B. (2004). Large-scale comparative genotyping and kinship analysis: Evolution in its use for human identification in mass fatality incidents and missing persons data basing. *Progress in Forensic Genetics, 10:*42–44.

McEvoy, K., and Conway, H. (2004). The dead, the law, and the politics of the past. *Journal of Law and Society, 31*(4):539–562.

MSF (Médecins Sans Frontières) (2006). *Living in fear: Colombia's cycle of violence.* http://www.msf.org

Nawrocki, S.P., Pless, J.E., Hawley, D.A., and Wagner, S.A. (1997). Fluvial transport of human crania. In *Forensic taphonomy: The postmortem fate of human remains,* Haglund, W.D., and Sorg, M.H. (Eds.). Boca Raton: CRC Press, pp. 529–552.

Owsley, D.W. (1995). Techniques for locating burials, with emphasis on the probe. *J. Forensic Sciences, 40:*735–740.

Pollack, C.E. (2003). Burial at Srebrenica: Linking place and trauma. *Social Science and Medicine, 56*(4):793–801.

Primorac, D., Andelinović, S., Definis-Govanić, M., Drmic, I., Rezic, B., Baden, M.M., Kennedy, M.A., Schanfield, M.S., Skakel, S.B., and Lee, H.C. (1996). Identification of war victims from mass graves in Croatia, Bosnia, and Herzegovina by the use of standard forensic methods and DNA typing. *J. Forensic Sciences, 41*(5):891–894.

Reichs, K.J. (1998). Postmortem dismemberment: Recovery, analysis and interpretation. In *Forensic osteology: Advances in the identification of human remains,* Reichs, K.J. (Ed.). Springfield: Charles C Thomas, pp. 353–388.

Reilley, B., and Morote, S. (2004). Caught in Colombia's crossfire. *The New England Journal of Medicine, 351*(25):2576–2578.

Samuelson, D.A., and Spirer, H.F. (1992). Use of incomplete and distorted data in inference about human rights violations. In *Human rights and statistics: Getting the record straight,* Jabine, T.B., and Claude, R.P. (Eds.). Philadelphia: University of Pennsylvania Press, pp. 62–77.

Schmitt, S. (2002). Mass graves and the collection of forensic evidence: Genocide, war crimes, and crimes against humanity. In *Advances in forensic taphonomy: Method, theory and archaeological perspectives,* Haglund, W.D., and Sorg, M.H. (Eds.). Boca Raton: CRC Press, pp. 277–292.

Silva, R., and Ball, P. (2006). *The profile of human rights violations in Timor-Leste, 1974–1999: A report by the Benetech human rights data analysis group to the commission on reception, truth and reconciliation.* http://www.hrdag.org/timor.

Simmons, T. (2002). Taphonomy of a karstic cave execution site at Hrgar, Bosnia-Herzegovina. In *Advances in forensic taphonomy: Method, theory and archaeological perspectives,* Haglund, W.D., and Sorg, M.H. (Eds.). Boca Raton: CRC Press, pp. 263–275.

Skinner, M. (1987). Planning the archaeological recovery of evidence from recent mass graves. *Forensic Science International, 34:*267–287.

Skinner, M., Alempijevic, D., and Djuric-Srejic, M. (2003). Guidelines for international forensic bio-archaeology monitors of mass grave exhumations. *Forensic Sci-*

ence International, 134:81–92.

Snow, C.C., and Bihurriet, M.J. (1992). An epidemiology of homicide: *Ningún nombre* burials in the Province of Buenos Aires from 1970 to 1984. In *Human rights and statistics: Getting the record straight,* Jabine, T.B., and Claude, R.P. (Eds.). Philadelphia: University of Pennsylvania Press, pp. 328–363.

Spennemann, D.H. and Franke, B. (1995). Archaeological techniques for exhumations: A unique data source for crime scene investigations. *Forensic Science International, 74*(1):5–15.

Steadman, D.L.W., and Haglund, W.D. (2005). The scope of anthropological contributions to human rights investigations. *J. Forensic Sciences, 50*(1):1–8.

Stover, E., Haglund, W.D., and Samuels, M. (2003). Exhumations of mass graves in Iraq: Considerations for forensic investigations, humanitarian needs, and the demands of justice. *Journal of the American Medical Association, 290*(5):663–66.

Stover, E., and Shigekane, R. (2002). The missing in the aftermath of war: When do the needs of victims' families and international war tribunals' clash? *International Review of the Red Cross, 84*(848):845–66.

Stover, E., and Shigekane, R. (2004). Exhumation of mass graves: Balancing legal and humanitarian needs. In *My neighbor, my enemy: Justice and community in the aftermath of mass atrocity,* Stover, E., and Weinstein, H.M. (Eds.). Cambridge: Cambridge University Press, pp. 85–103.

Summerfield, D. (1995). Addressing human response to war and atrocity. In *Beyond trauma: Cultural and societal dynamics,* Kleber, F.C., and Gersons, B. (Eds.). New York: Plenum Press, pp. 17–29.

Symes, S.A., Williams, J.A., Murray, E.A., Hoffman, J.M., Holland, T.D., Saul, J.M., Saul, F.P., and Pope, E.J. (2002). Taphonomic context of sharp-force trauma in suspected cases of human mutilation and dismemberment. In *Advances in forensic taphonomy: Method, theory, and archaeological perspectives,* Haglund, W.D., and Sorg, M.H. (Eds.). Boca Raton: CRC Press, pp. 403–434.

UNWGEID (United Nations Working Group on Enforced or Involuntary Disappearances) (2006). *Mission to Colombia.* E/CN.4/2006/56/Add.1, January 17.

Chapter 9

FORENSIC ARCHAEOLOGY AND THE SCIENTIFIC DOCUMENTATION OF HUMAN RIGHTS VIOLATIONS: AN ARGENTINIAN EXAMPLE FROM THE EARLY 1980s

PATRICIA BERNARDI AND LUIS FONDEBRIDER

INTRODUCTION

Within the modern context, it is commonplace to discuss the uses of forensic archaeology and forensic anthropology in the framework of human rights investigations. Since 1996, when the International Criminal Tribunal for the former Yugoslavia (ICTY) began a program of forensic investigations on a number of mass graves situated across the former Yugoslavia, with a particular emphasis on Bosnia, many scientists have devoted themselves to work in applying those disciplines to human rights investigations.

The effectiveness of the different techniques and excavation methods utilized has been proven, ensuring that forensic archaeology is now an essential element of medicolegal investigations (United Nations, 1991; Doretti and Snow, 2003; Skinner and Sterenberg, 2005; Skinner et al., 2003; Haglund, 2001; Fondebrider, 2004). This relationship, of course, is observed not only in human rights investigations, but also within the routine of day-to-day police work in many countries.

Twenty years ago, in 1987, it was necessary to begin a forensic investigation in Argentina, pertaining to a series of mass graves containing the remains of many of the victims who had disappeared during the last military government (1976–1983). The task seemed of unbounded extent and, furthermore, completely new. At that time, archaeologists, not only in Argentina, but in most countries around the world, were not accustomed to taking part in forensic exhumations, nor were forensic anthropologists involved in analyzing and identifying remains found within this type of context (Doretti and Snow, 2003; Fondebrider, 2005). Resultantly, at that juncture, many diverse questions arose from those who were becoming involved for the first time in human rights investigations, and were facing new circumstances, including:

- Is it possible to conduct this type of research within a country in which democratic foundations have not been firmly established?
- Is it safe to participate in an investigation of this type, while those responsible for the crimes are still at liberty?
- How will the judicial sector deal with the fact that processing such graves may take several months, or even years to accomplish?
- Will the financial resources be adequate enough to carry such tasks through to completion?
- How might requests posed by the victims' relatives to be present during excavations be sensitively dealt with?
- Is it reasonable to utilize techniques that would be applied within the context of archaeological sites that are hundreds of years old?
- Is it preferable to remove the bodies from the ground as soon as they are uncovered, or after the entire grave has been exposed?
- Should the skeletal remains be left on a pedestal?
- Is it feasible to rely on ballistic analyses that may be performed by the same security forces that committed the crimes that are being investigated?

Such issues, and many others, as odd as they may seem, are to be confronted with when investigating any deaths related to political violence.

It is completely different to work under the umbrella of the United Nations, as in the case of the International Criminal Tribunal for the former Yugoslavia (ICTY), or to have the support of the world's leading countries, such as the International Commission on Missing Persons (ICMP), also within the Yugoslavian context. Such bodies, as the United Nations, provide the political, financial, judicial, and security context, as well as the necessary infrastructure that are prerequisites for such enormous tasks to be effectively undertaken. Resultantly, this leaves the forensic archaeologist with only the task of concentrating on his/her work: to excavate the grave(s) by the most effective means possible, recovering the remains in an adequate manner, at a reasonable pace, and causing a minimal amount of damage to any evidence that might be present. It is within this context, exceptional in almost all aspects, that many forensic investigators, from a variety of disciplines, have been trained, making it difficult for them, sometimes, to work in other settings.

Unfortunately, such kinds of facilitations are rarely guaranteed. Amidst all the regions which have suffered from political violence, only the former Yugoslavia has received boundless, unceasing political and economical support from the United Nations, as well as from the world's leading countries. Such international support has been much needed in order to facilitate forensic investigations which aim to exhume and identify the remains of the thousands of victims of human rights violations that occurred in that particular area.

From 1996 until the present, hundreds of millions of dollars have been invested in the former Yugoslavia to fund forensic investigations. But in the rest of the world, in many countries such as Rwanda, El Salvador, Indonesia, Democratic Republic of Congo (DRC) or Cambodia, just to mention a few examples, thousands of families are still waiting to recover the remains of their murdered relatives, even when, in many cases, the locations of the graves containing the remains of their loved ones are widely acknowledged.

After 23 years of experience in the field of human rights investigations, and having worked in 34 countries throughout the world, the members of the Argentine Forensic Anthropology Team (EAAF) have arrived at the conclusion that, aside from the technical difficulties that may arise during prospecting, excavating and analyzing graves, in a large number of cases, there are also a variety of other political, judicial, psychological, economic and logistical problems that should be born in mind prior to undertaking such investigations, since these factors may severely affect the task at hand. Some of these elements include:

- The lack of political support from the new government of the country where the investigations are to be conducted.
- A lack of legal authority that will approve the investigation of a grave.
- The grave being held under the custody of those who may actually be responsible for the crimes committed.

- The lack of a budget adequate enough to provide security staff.
- The lack of a legal framework that would allow forensic archaeologists and anthropologists to take part in the exhumation and analysis of the recovered remains, instead of the tasks being assigned to local medical doctors or criminalists.
- The distrust that may exist on behalf of the families of the victims towards the governmental representatives undertaking the investigations.
- A lack of security in the area in which the graves are situated, because of the absence of State authority or the unwillingness to perform its role.
- The mishandling of evidence recovered, and the lack of security pertaining to its custody.
- The fear of possible reprisals against witnesses.
- The lack of a budget adequate enough to carry through the investigation to a satisfactory conclusion.

Additionally, it is of great importance to take into account that the majority of the abducted individuals, who are tortured and murdered as victims of political violence around the globe, principally belong to lower social stratums. They usually reside outside of the main cities, within areas in which the government exerts little or no influence; as a consequence, graves may not be situated within areas of easy access, and basic services may be largely absent.

A comprehensive investigation may demand an investment in infrastructure and logistics, as well as in security frameworks, which for reasons already stated, may not be forthcoming, and which may resultantly serve to effect an inadequate investigation, or the prospect of one not being attempted at all.

Moreover, it may come to pass that the actual investigators may belong to a partially or even totally different culture to that of the victims and their relatives. This may occur when specialists arrive from the city to work in the countryside, but it is particularly true when the investigators travel to work in a foreign country of which they may have little knowledge, culturally or socially (reference is made to such issues in Chapter 10 of this volume).

Furthermore, the families of the victims don't always share the wishes or objectives of the judicial authorities, and as a result, local traditions and religious beliefs may not be respected. A careless exhumation, unaware of the relatives' desires, may ignore the rituals regarding transit from life to death, which may be a prerequisite to ensure that the victim will rest in peace and have access to his or her own place in the cosmos.

All the above mentioned circumstances that affect the conditions of this type of forensic work makes it impossible to create generalizations beforehand. The forensic investigations in the former Yugoslavia can be used as a guide in some aspects, particularly in dealing with recent big mass graves, commingled remains, and other particular issues, but in many other aspects it is not possible to replicate in most of the countries where these kinds of investigations are necessary. It is not a model that can be transported and installed as a factory, producing exhumations and identifications, and it would be a mistake, for example, to confuse the situation in the former Yugoslavia with the situation in Iraq (see Chapters 7 and 11 respectively in this volume), just to mention some of the countries where different scientists have been involved during the last two years performing exhumations.

Among the few organizations working in the field of forensic anthropology and human rights, the Guatemalan Forensic Anthropology Foundation (FAFG), and the Argentine Forensic Anthropology Team (EAAF) (the authors being members of the latter) are distinct from other organizations dealing with investigations related to this field in a number of different aspects:

- The members themselves belong to countries which were affected by political violence, the reason why they are knowledgeable with the respective contexts.
- They are both independent, non-profit organizations with scientific objectives.
- Their members are professionals with full-time dedication to their duties.
- Not only do their members perform the exhumations and analysis of the recovered remains, but they also carry out an investigation previous to each case, consisting of interviews with witnesses and victim's relatives, gathering antemortem data, etc.
- They have their own laboratories devoted to anthropological analysis.
- Young people who become part of these organizations have the opportunity of receiving training by working on real mass graves and studying contemporary skeletons.

- There is a close and positive connection with human rights organizations composed of relatives of the victims.
- The EAAF in particular has enriched its experience as a result of having worked in more than 30 countries all over the world, within diverse cultural, political, juridical and religious environments.
- The FAFG has investigated, since 1992, thousands of cases in Guatemala, the Latin American country which suffered the greatest volume of disappearances and massacres as performed by successive governments. At the present time, the FAFG have exhumed hundreds of common graves, and have also carried through the analysis of thousands of recovered skeletal remains, having to deal, in the process, with a variety of technical difficulties.

These characteristics, some of which are shared by other institutions or individuals committed to forensic anthropology in Latin America, are the reasons why the investigations related to human rights violations may vary, depending on their specific context, who the researchers are, and what type of relationship they hold to the victim's relatives.

THE ARGENTINIAN CASE (1976–1983)

On March 24th, 1976 the constitutional government of Isabel Perón was overthrown by the means of a coup d'état headed by the Armed Forces, an action consistent with a tradition of military governments that had begun in Argentina in 1930. But on this occasion, it was different: a policy of state terrorism was put into effect, resulting in the abduction and disappearance of at least 10,000 people, although human rights groups give higher figures.

In 1983, democracy was reinstated through the election of a new government. By then, thousands of relatives wanted to know the whereabouts of the disappeared; they desired information that would clarify what had actually happened to their loved ones, and their demand had a strong influence upon the restoration of democracy. In response, the new government attempted to provide answers in a variety of different ways, including the creation of a Truth Commission, known as the National Commission on the Disappeared (CONADEP), and by passing a legal judgment on those who were responsible for the "disappearances."

Thus, the disappearance and murder of thousands of victims, formerly denounced by human rights organizations, was being confirmed.

Abductees were typically imprisoned within one of the hundreds of Clandestine Detention Centers (CDCs) commanded and administered by the police and Armed Forces. Once imprisoned, such individuals were tortured and, in most cases, extra-judicially executed by shooting. Their remains were then buried in unmarked graves, but often in specific areas of many municipal cemeteries throughout the country. However, some CDCs disposed of many of the victims by sedating them, the bodies then being bound and thrown from military aircraft into rivers or into the Argentine Sea. Approximately 60 of these bodies were later recovered, having washed up onto the Argentinian and Uruguayan coasts. In those days, the military government denied the existence of any disappeared individuals, and the families were never informed of their fate.

During 1984, along with the reinstatement of democracy arose the possibility of investigating the burials of the unidentified victims. Exhumations and analysis of the bodies were required in order to establish their identities and the causes of their deaths, information that was to subsequently be transformed into legal evidence.

Initially, the judicial authorities searching for the remains of the disappeared employed the existing forensic services. Unfortunately, this meant that neither archaeologists nor anthropologists were involved in the exhumations; this task was instead carried out by gravediggers and firemen with no special training. Similarly, the subsequent studies of the recovered human remains were carried out by forensic scientists lacking experience in the analysis of skeletal remains. As a result, several of the remains recovered were destroyed, important evidence was lost, and few victims were subsequently identified.

Under such circumstances, it became clear that a more formal approach was required and that working methods would have to change. The CONADEP and the Grandmothers of the Plaza de Mayo, a local human rights organization, requested assistance from the Science and Human Rights program, part of the American Association for the Advancement of Science (AAAS), based in Washington, DC. In 1984, this organization assembled a delegation of seven forensic experts to visit Argentina. Among them was Dr. Clyde Snow, an eminent forensic anthropologist, who in the 1970s began to employ archaeologists in the recovery of skeletal remains (Doretti and Fondebrider, 2004). Dr. Snow was the first forensic anthropologist to apply the discipline of forensic anthropology to the analysis of victims of large scale human rights violations, and within the context of political violence.[1] Dr. Snow, after his initial participation, remained in Argentina for several years, during which time he trained the current members of the EAAF (Snow, 1984a; Snow, 1984b; Snow and Bihurriet, 1992).

THE COMMON GRAVES IN THE AVELLANEDA CEMETERY, PROVINCE OF BUENOS AIRES

Background

During October 1986, the office of the Prosecutor who was conducting the trial against the military authorities, requested the EAAF to perform an urgent forensic exhumation with the correct archaeological techniques on Sector 134, an area located within the Avellaneda Cemetery, in close proximity to the cemetery's morgue, and located in a densely populated zone in the southern part of Buenos Aires Province, 12 km from the Federal Capital of Buenos Aires.

During the hearings that were being held as part of the trial, a former officer during the dictatorship had claimed that Rafael Perrota, a journalist who had directed *El Cronista Comercial*, a local newspaper, and who had been kidnapped in July 1977, had been buried in that sector. Due to this information, an investigation was urgently requested.

With the available information being so imprecise, it was decided before initial exhumation to fathom an area of 2 m × 1 m, following the instructions of one of the gravediggers. It was promptly discovered that the site contained a common grave, thus making it necessary to dig the entire area, so as to carry out a comprehensive search. After receiving

---

1. After this experience, exhumations were carried out in Chile, in 1989, with the creation of the Chilean Forensic Anthropology Group (GAF). In 1992, with the creation of the Guatemalan Forensic Anthropology Team, exhumations began in Central America in a massive way. In 1993, the first exhumations were undertaken in Croatia by a team assembled by Physicians for Human Rights, through the United Nations Commission of Experts, comprised of Argentinian, Chilean, Guatemalan and American anthropologists. In Iraq, a similar team in 1992 had already begun to investigate the attacks perpetrated by Hussein's government against the Kurds. In 1994, the EAAF began to work in various areas of Africa, such as Ethiopia, South Africa, Zimbabwe and the Democratic Republic of the Congo (DRC). In such a manner, the young Argentinian, Chilean and Guatemalan scientists joined together by Dr. Snow, pioneered the application of forensic sciences to the documentation of human rights violations, known, since 1996, as "Forensic Anthropology and Human Rights."

the corresponding report, the Court allowed the EAAF to excavate the entire sector. This task commenced in 1988.

Sector 134

Sector 134 is a rectangular area (12 m × 24 m, containing a total area of 288 sq. m) located at the back of the Avellaneda Cemetery, placed between the main graveyard and a city street. A 2 meter high brick wall, built after the military coup, isolated Sector 134, with a small gate providing access to the rest of the cemetery. On the east side, it was bordered by a building that served as a morgue and storage area for cadavers.

A gate present in the street side wall was wide enough to allow vehicles to enter the cemetery. The solid metal gates and high walls concealed the cemetery from the eyes of curious passers-by. During the first three years of the dictatorship, during which thousands of people disappeared, neighbors across the street observed military trucks and police vehicles entering Sector 134 through the street-side gate day and night.

After 1982, Sector 134 seemed to have been abandoned, and it gradually became overgrown with weeds. Although it was suspected that it concealed remains of some of those who had disappeared, this area, like similar places in Argentina, could not be investigated until after 1983, when democracy was reinstated (Doretti and Snow, 2003).

In 1998, when the EAAF commenced their investigation in Sector 134, the challenge was enormous. From the technical point of view, there were almost no forensic cases in the world that could exemplify how to work with several mass graves within a context of human rights violations. At the same time, there was ample information about the bodies buried in Sector 134, but the data came from several sources, and neither the judges nor the lawyers were interested in taking on the task of collecting all the information, analyzing it and developing hypotheses relating to the location of the bodies and their identities.

It was clear that forensic work in Sector 134 went beyond the usual routine of exhuming the remains, trying to identify them and establishing their cause and manner of death. The Avellaneda Cemetery provided us with an opportunity to study the bureaucratic machinery of the repression through the layers of evidence it generated. As is quite usual when the State is the body organizing the repression, despite all the secrecy surrounding the abduction, illegal detention, torturing and killing of people, once the bodies were disposed of in public places, a whole chain of bureaucratic steps followed. Thus, many official documents were generated, such as autopsy records, fingerprints, death certificates, cemetery records, burial certificates, among others, all of which are vital in these types of investigations.

At this point, during the first years of activity of the EAAF, it became evident that the exhumation and analysis of recovered remains could not be independent of a much needed historical research, pertaining to each case. Consequently, all written and oral sources related to Sector 134 began to be investigated, as well as reported disappearances in the surrounding areas between 1976 and 1983.

The Historical Research

During the preliminary historical research, which always precedes and often continues during the archaeological phase, the EAAF searched for death and burial certificates in the Avellaneda Cemetery records and surrounding registry offices. These records illustrated that, despite all the secrecy surrounding the repression, at least 245 people were recorded as being buried in Sector 134 during the era of the military government, with each individual possessing a death certificate. Of these individuals, 160 were ascertained as being young people who had been killed by gunshot wounds, and brought there by police or military personnel. The majority of all of the bodies were buried between 1976 and 1977 (96 individuals and 110 individuals, respectively) during the peak of the repression, decreasing sharply from 1978 onwards (only 6 individuals being buried that year) until 1982.

Based on the data available, and on our own historical research, EAAF approached Sector 134 with a series of hypotheses as to what might be discovered there. In view that the typical method employed by the Argentine army when disposing of the bodies of the disappeared was to bury them as NN (no name) in public cemeteries, Snow and Bihurriet (1992) conducted a statistical study in 1984, based on cemetery and registry office records, covering large sectors of the regions most affected by the repression, including "normal" and military government years. The study showed a clear shift in the biological and traumatic profile of the NN population during military governmental rule. Usually, in "normal" years, this population was generally represented by older individuals, mostly men, who had died from "natural" causes such as neglect, old age, sometimes exposure, malnutrition, and frequently due to alcohol abuse. Their remains were usually brought to the cemetery by hospices and hospitals, firefighters, and police. According to Snow and Bihurriet (1992), depending largely on the size of the population it serves, a municipal cemetery can expect a fairly constant annual number of NN burials. This number may show transitory peaks related to mass disasters and longer term upward or downward trends related to population growth or economic factors influencing poverty rates and homelessness, but, usually, it remains fairly stable for a given cemetery.

However, the NN population from the period of the military government was very different. Firstly, there was a statistically significant increase in the number of NNs per year in a number of cemeteries within crucial areas most hit by the repression, such as the cemeteries surrounding the city of Buenos Aires. Secondly, in these cemeteries, the biological profile of the NNs had changed. The majority was now comprised of young people between 20 and 35 years of age, with women representing approximately 30 percent of the total amount, illustrating an important increase in the traditional NN female population. The cause of death for most of these young individuals was violent, mostly due to gunshot wounds. They were often brought to the cemetery by military or police personnel. All these patterns are consistent with those seen among the disappeared (Snow and Bihurriet, 1992).

Information collected by CONADEP during 1984 revealed that 80 percent of the reported disappearances were registered between 1976 and 1977; 30 percent of the almost 10,000 disappeared individuals were women, and 70 percent of the victims were between 21 and 35 years of age at the time of death.

The strong correlation with the population described in Snow and Bihurriet's study (1992), in terms of age, sex, and cause of death, lent weight to the claim that Sector 134 was the final burial site to a large percentage of many disappeared and executed individuals.

In this case, the sheer quantity of relevant information, and the way in which it was fragmented among many sources, meant that several months had to be devoted to preliminary work before initiating the exhumations. Even so, because we never cease to receive and compile relevant facts, the "preliminary" phase remains an ongoing one.

However, the individual identification of the remains presented a much more complicated problem. The system of repression was complex in Argentina. Prisoners could pass through several of the more than 350 CDCs identified throughout the country by the CONADEP in 1984. The possible combinations and permutations of this process were potentially enormous, making the task of tracing the journey of a given *desaparecido* (disappeared individual), from his or her place of abduction to his or her grave, a formidable problem. Fortunately, however, patterns of modality emerged among the security forces, even though each force and paramilitary group had their own modalities that could also vary over the years during the dictatorship, and from region to region. Part of EAAF's work in Argentina is to reconstruct this *modus operandi* through documents and interviews with survivors.

EAAF collected and examined among other sources, judicial, police, and military files, relatives' reports, and the testimonies of survivors of CDCs; such details provided important information that was pertinent when investigating Sector 134, where prisoner's bodies had been disposed of.

Initially, we consulted materials from a judicial case relating to irregularities in the manner burials had been dealt with in Sector 134. Next, we tracked in *La Opinión* newspaper all the reports concerning armed confrontations, or discoveries of unidentified bodies between 1975 and 1979. In this manner, we attempted to establish connections among alleged shootouts between security forces and guerrilla groups, the discoveries of bodies, and burials at Sector 134 in the Avellaneda Cemetery.

We also consulted materials from judicial and military files that could be related to the Avellaneda Cemetery. Files containing valuable information about the discovery of unidentified bodies that were later buried in Sector 134 were located. These files had dates of findings and general physical information about the victims, useful for correlating with information on "transfers," a euphemism used by security forces to refer to the moment when prisoners were taken from their last CDC to be killed. Unfortunately, the dates on which these individuals were last seen alive is only approximate, and we have no information about the actual dates of death. Some of the files also contained autopsy reports produced by physicians attached to police forces soon after the bodies were discovered, in addition to fingerprints, and in some cases, photographs of the actual bodies were available.

A key source of information was the *"Deaths"* archive from the Provincial Person's Registry, from which we gathered information from all death certificates concerning unidentified cadavers and those killed by violent or suspicious means in Buenos Aires Province between 1976 and 1978. Among these were additional death certificates linked to burials in Avellaneda Cemetery, as well as certificates linked to all the southern municipalities close to Avellaneda (Lanús, Quilmes, Lomas de Zamora,

Almirante Brown, Florencio Varela, Berazategui, La Plata, Ensenada, and Berisso). As part of this task, we gathered all the available death certificates, 245 in total, concerning those buried in Sector 134.

Finally, we incorporated survivors' reports and other information pertinent to individuals observed in nearby CDCs. The EAAF also collected information pertaining to the members of union, political, student and guerrilla groups who were primary targets for persecution during those years. When the kidnappers made "sweeps" targeting a particular group, their members were likely to end up in the same CDCs and eventually, in the same burial sites.

Based on this previous investigation, EAAF started to collect ante-mortem data or physical information provided by families, dentists and medical doctors, about the disappeared who could potentially have been buried in Sector 134. This allowed us to compile dossiers on the alleged victims. Crucial preliminary information pertaining to such individuals included the time of death or disappearance, sex, height, dental information, and reports of old injuries, among other details, which are sometimes important keys in effecting positive identifications. In addition, genealogical information and blood samples are often collected from the surviving relatives of victims for eventual DNA analysis. Collecting all this information may require several interviews with family members over a period of months or years. With patience and sensitivity, bonds of trust and understanding are built with the families, making it easier for them to recover and piece together their lives as affected by events from a painful past.

When possible, we also try to reconstruct the final days of those who were killed, so that we can create hypotheses pertaining to their fates, and where their remains may be located. Additionally, we try to provide this information to the victims' families, who often desire to obtain every piece of available information relating to their beloved ones.

THE ARCHAEOLOGICAL EXCAVATION

Planning the Excavation

Every excavation presents challenges of its own. The criteria that one is confronted with are specific to each case, but take into consideration certain general rules. There are some factors that should always be borne in mind; the physical environment, the size of the area in question, the possible number of remains to be exhumed and, foremost, what type of information one is most likely to uncover (Ubelaker, 1989).

The objective of an excavation is to find out as exactly as possible the manner and conditions in which the remains were first interred. Nevertheless, to identify their precise location and depth is also an essential part of the research (Morse et al., 1983; Sigler-Eisenberg, 1985; Skinner, 1987; Ferllini Timms, 1993; France et al., 1992; Haglund, 2001; Haglund and Sorg, 1997; Haglund et al., 2001; Hunter et al., 1996; Hunter et al., 2001).

EAAF began exhumations at the Avellaneda Cemetery in 1988, concluding these during 1992, once the entire area had been comprehensively excavated. Although the data from the judicial file and other written sources was full of gaps, it did indicate that some nineteen common graves were dug in Sector 134 between April 1976 and September 1978.

Cleaning and Preparation of the Area

One of the first tasks to accomplish, so as to properly plan the excavation, especially bearing in mind the preliminary steps of the investigation, was to carefully remove overgrown vegetation from the area, and to accurately define the sector's topography. The area was cleaned manually, using machetes and shovels to cut the vegetation and collect rubbish that lay on the field (Fig. 9-1). After doing so, it was possible to

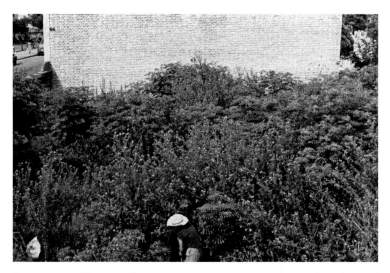

Figure 9-1. Cleaning Sector 134 in preparation for archaeological intervention.

discern an unevenness of the surface of the ground, seemingly caused by the inhumations (Fig. 9-2). This effect was organized into two parallel axes, over the east and west side respectively.

Taking into account the extent of the field, (almost 300 sq. m), and the number of remains to be recovered, a quadrille scheme of the sector was elaborated. The ground was divided into 41 excavation units or quadrants of 2.50 m × 2.50 m, with a path of 0.50 m between each of them. A Cartesian coordinates' scheme was designed, with one of its axes named with letters and the other with numbers (Fig. 9-3).

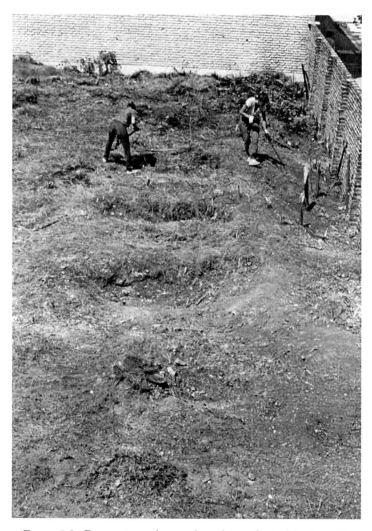

Figure 9-2. Depressions observed on the surface of Sector 134.

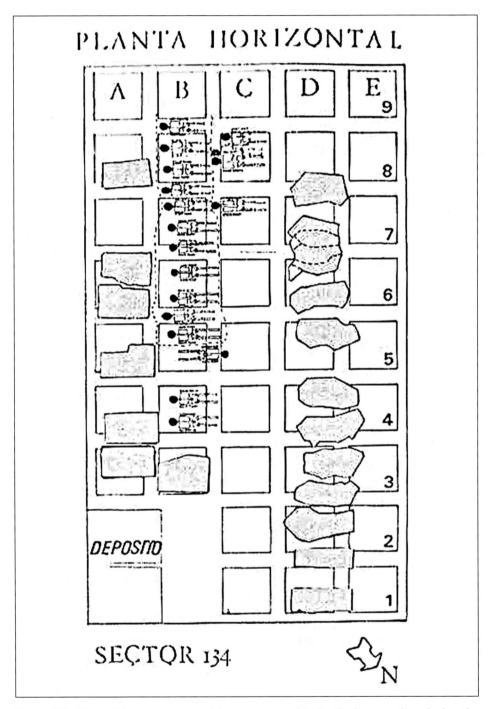

Figure 9-3. Plan of the excavation with common and individual graves found after the digging was completed.

Ground level was fixed at 0.75 m from the surface, and was designated by the means of a yellow stripe painted onto the walls of Sector 134. From that point, the depth in which the remains laid was measured. Within each unit, an excavation was performed respecting the natural layers of the ground, attempting to discover the original boundaries of the grave.

During the first year, labor was focused upon the west area, corresponding to row "D" of the diagram (Fig. 9-3). Initially, skeletons were left there in order to appreciate the relationships between them, and within the context of Sector 134; this was decided upon because it would provide a more complete picture of the finds to the judges. This also served to effect an efficient utilization of the area. However, the remains in question were later removed for reasons of climate and security.

Archaeologically speaking, there were two kinds of burial sites present in the area, individual and common graves; both types were considered to constitute primary graves. Within common graves, we discovered two basic types, "synchronic" and "diachronic." Synchronic graves are those in which the bodies seem to have been deposited at the same time, since there are no observable elements separating the bodies (Fig. 9-4). Diachronic graves are those in which bodies seem to have been deposited at different times, a conclusion based, in this case, upon the earth layers separating the different layers of corpses (Fig. 9-5).

According to the cemetery records, the most plausible scenario would seem to be that bodies were transferred from the morgue to the graves, usually in groups, and then covered, with the earth not reaching the surface level of the ground. In this manner, another layer of bodies might be deposited there after a period of a week, several months or a year. This resulted in a stratigraphy of levels, in which the skeletal remains were separated by layers of compacted earth. As the exhumations proceeded, we observed precisely such a pattern.

The results of reuse and layering can be illustrated by imagining a vertical cross-section of the quadrant designated D6/7 (Fig. 9-3). By viewing the section from the side, we could observe that there had been two episodes of burial. The first skeleton discovered in that quadrant was buried at a depth of 26 cm. After removing it, we found a layer of earth 75 cm deep, and then a second group of skeletons. Unfortunately, since they are very recent, the two layers cannot be dated by the same means used to date ancient burials, such as the Carbon-14 method. Such methods are also not useful when trying to establish short-term

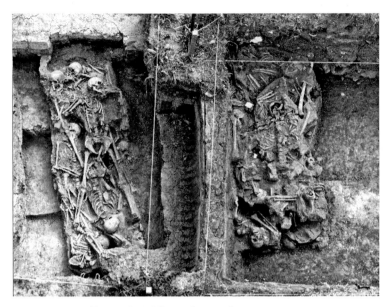

Figure 9-4. View of a synchronic grave.

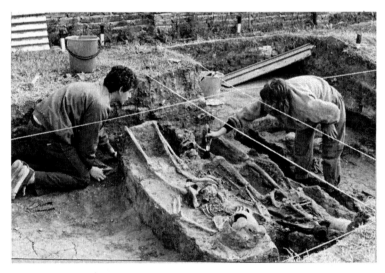

Figure 9-5. Work being conducted on a diachronic grave.

differences in time, as probably one layer was a week, a month or a few years older than the other. However, we can establish relative sequences, that is, that the lower level is older than the one closer to the surface, and work toward hypotheses pertaining to the time that had elapsed between the episodes of burial.

Archaeological Findings

Through careful archaeological work, the team was able to expose the graves and carefully record its findings (see Figure 9-6 a-e). Once the work had been concluded, the team had obtained a much clearer picture of Sector 134. As follows is a list of these findings:

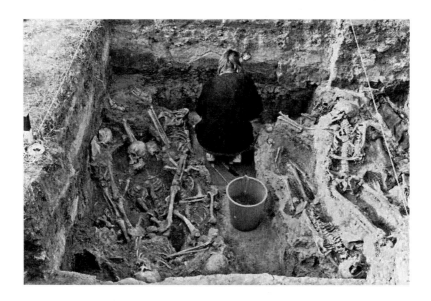

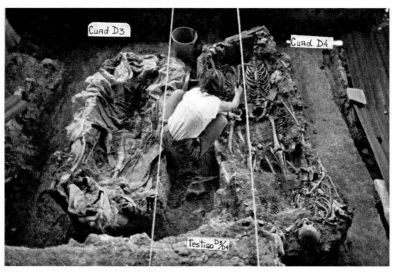

Figure 9-6 a–b. A general view of some of the graves with the skeletons already exposed.

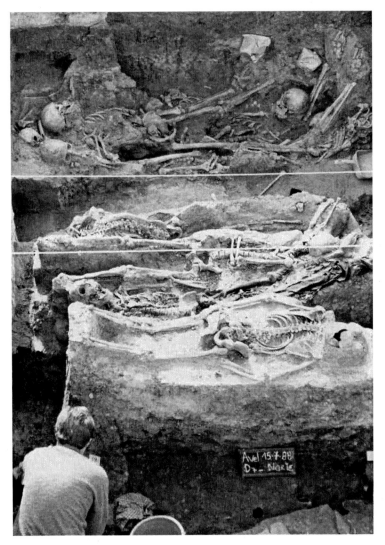

Figure 9-6 c. A general view of some of the graves with the skeletons already exposed.

- Three hundred and thirty-six skeletons were exhumed from Sector 134, 91 more bodies than registered in the records of the cemetery.
- The remains were deposited within 18 individual graves and 19 common graves.
- Fifteen common graves were synchronic, and the other 4 were diachronic (quadrants D6/7, D5, A4 and A5), (Fig. 9-3). Although layers of earth were mingled between the different inhumations in

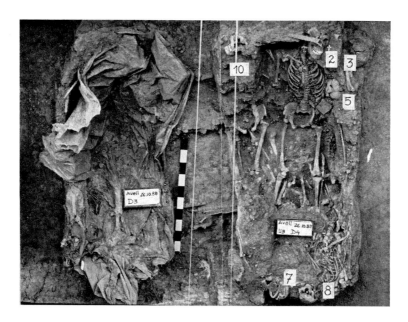

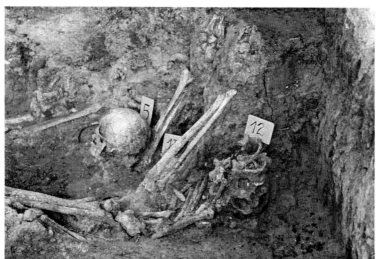

Figure 9-6 d–e. A general view of some of the graves with the skeletons already exposed.

the diachronic graves, the characteristics of the area made it impossible to determine the period of time between them.
• Three hundred and twenty-two of the skeletons had an anatomic layout. This meant that the bodies were deposited while still possessing soft tissue, the reason why they remained in a certain position.

- The minimum amount of recovered skeletons in common graves was 3 (grave D1), and the greatest amount was 28 (grave D2/3).
- The deepest grave was D8, reaching 210 cm in depth.
- With the exception of two skeletons discovered in graves D8 and D5, all bodies were oriented from east to west, confirming the data provided by the gravediggers.
- Only 30 percent of the individuals exhibited remnants of clothing, with personal effects being very rare. Wedding rings were found among the hand bones of two individuals and metal crosses associated with two others. Three coins, one dated 1958, and the other two 1976, were also recovered.
- Ballistic evidence consisted of more than 300 bullet fragments; no cartridge cases were discovered.

Laboratory Work: Anthropological Analysis

The laboratory phase commenced during mid-1991, and was focused on the anthropological analysis of the 336 skeletons exhumed from Sector 134. Initially, we set up a makeshift lab in an old morgue of the Avellaneda Cemetery. Subsequently, in April, 2000, the Court authorized us to move the skeletons to our own laboratory at EAAF's offices.

The first step of the study consisted of selective x-raying, which was concentrated on bones exhibiting any suspicious lesions. Teeth and bone samples were preserved for future DNA analysis; afterwards, we cleaned and labeled the skeletons. Finally, we reconstructed and glued together fractured pieces.

After these basic preparations, we could begin to make the essential observations and measurements for each individual, in order to obtain a biological profile. We made careful records of all pathologies and wounds observable in the skeletal remains. Finally, we codified basic information about each individual's dentition, and took photographs of both the upper and lower teeth. All of this information was incorporated into the individual's dossier and stored in a searchable database (Buikstra and Ubelaker, 1994; Grauer, 1995; Workshop of European Anthropologists, 1980; Fondebrider and Mendoca, 2001; Rodríguez, 1994).

EAAF's database consists of seven screens, each corresponding to one of the estimations or determinations carried out in the laboratory. This format makes it easy to consult, to conduct searches, and to generate statistics about populations by the means of features. For example, one could quickly determine the number of female skeletons between the ages 18 to 22, or the number of male skeletons with statures greater than or equal to 180 cm.

Following the laboratory analysis, we attempted to move towards the identification of the remains.

Sex and Age Distributions

The number of bodies exhumed from Sector 134 exceeded the number of those recorded in the cemetery registry by 91 individuals, the difference being composed mainly of 77 male skeletons. Table 9-1 shows a comparison of sex distribution between the skeletons actually recovered from Sector 134, and also according to the cemetery's registry. Skeletons in the "undetermined" category include those belonging to prepubescent children, and some that were incomplete.

TABLE 9-1. COMPARISON BETWEEN THE DISTRIBUTION BY SEX AND

	Male	*Female*	*Undetermined*	*Totals*
Exhumed skeletons	252 indiv. **75%**	71 indiv. **21.1%**	13 indiv. **3.9%**	336 indiv.
Cemetery records	175 indiv. **71.4%**	53 indiv. **21.6%**	17 indiv. **7%**	245 indiv.

TOTAL NUMBER OF BODIES EXHUMED TO THOSE LISTED IN THE
CEMETERY RECORDS FROM SECTOR 134

The age distribution for the bodies exhumed ranged from fetuses to those over 50 years of age, representing a wide age range (see Table 9-2). The first group was comprised of thirteen individuals aged 13 and under at the time of death. Among them, one individual, Carlos Manfil, was identified by the use of mitochondrial DNA testing, this individual being eight years old at the time of death. The other was a 12-year-old girl, who was already identified, but not related to a disappearance. Seven corresponded to newborns, and four to fetuses. Of this last group, the ages indicated are between 9–10 lunar months and 1–1.5 years. None of the skeletal remains compatible with newborns were found in direct associations with female adult skeletons.

Of the skeletons recovered from Sector 134, the largest concentration is in the 21 to 35 age group, with 135 skeletons, or 40.1 percent (Table 9-2). This coincides with the age distribution of the population as described by Snow and Bihurriet (1992) in their demographic study of people that disappeared during Argentina's "Dirty War."

The next largest concentration is in the over 50 category, with a total of 108 individuals, or 32.1 percent of the remains recovered from Sector 134 (Table 9-2). Fifty-two persons registered in the cemetery record books form part of this concentration. In terms of sex, age, and cause of death, this group coincides closely with the profile of the indigent population. Nevertheless, it is significant that eleven individuals in the over 50 age group exhibited bullet wounds.

Age group	0-13 years	14-20 years	21-35 years	36-50 years	Over 50 years	Undeter- mined	Totals
Exhumed Individuals	13	15	135	58	108	7	336
Percentages	3.9%	4.5%	40.1%	17.3%	32.1%	2.1%	100%

TABLE 9-2. THE BODIES' AGE DISTRIBUTION FROM SECTOR 134

Thus, the overall pattern is indicative of the fact that during the six years that Sector 134 was in use (1976–1982), the bodies of "ordinary people" (mostly elderly male indigents) were buried in the same mass graves as the *desaparecidos* (disappeared), who were predominately young, and often, female.

Cause of Death

Many injuries related to causes of death leave no trace in skeletal remains. For this reason, sometimes the cause of death must be left as "undetermined." Furthermore, even in cases in which sufficient trauma to cause the death of an individual was identified in a skeleton, other elements may also have contributed to, or even caused, the death of a person, and are no longer available, as they only affected the soft tissue. In Sector 134, among the traumatic causes of death, we recorded evidence of gunshot wounds, and cases of partially or totally burned skeletons (DiMaio, 1985). Among those classified as "undetermined" are skeletons found incomplete and/or disarticulated, and those of newborns, infants, and fetuses (Table 9-3).

	With perimortem lesions	Without perimortem lesions	Undetermined	Totals
Totals	178	133	25	336
Percentages	**53%**	**39.6%**	**7.4%**	**100%**

TABLE 9-3. DISTRIBUTION OF THE EXHUMED SKELETONS ACCORDING TO THE CAUSE OF DEATH FROM SECTOR 134

Evidence of gunshot wounds to the head and/or to the chest was present in 178 individuals (53 percent) of the total, almost all of whom were under 50 years of age at the time of death. Conversely, gunshot wounds are rare in the over fifty age group. Some of the other younger individuals exhibited blunt force trauma and burning; others within the same group showed no signs of gunshot wounds, burning and/or blunt force trauma; however, they may have also died violently, since it is known that a number of the disappeared died due to physical torture (mostly electric shocks) that would not leave marks on the bones.

In sum, the remains exhumed at Sector 134 illustrate the two groups of NNs discussed at the beginning of this section: an older one, in which most individuals show no signs of violent cause of death, very likely representing the "normal" or "traditional" population of NNs, and a younger one, illustrating in most cases a violent cause of death, mostly by gunshot wounds, very likely corresponding to the *desaparecido* group. This distribution and features are consistent with Snow and Bihurriet's study (1992).

Identification

Another interesting feature observed with reference to the remains from Sector 134 was that sixteen showed evidence, mostly in the skulls, of having been autopsied. Although it was standard procedure for local authorities to perform an autopsy when a body was unidentified, and/or whenever the cause of death was violent, suspicious, or unattended, the practice of these autopsies was remarkable, given the way that the bodies were treated afterwards.

Of the 336 skeletons recovered, ten presented saw marks to the distal part of the forearms, but the hand bones were not recovered. This was the result of a standard procedure of the Buenos Aires Provincial Police until the 1970s. When bodies were discovered in public places, they would often sever the hands and send them to their dactyloscopy laboratory for fingerprinting, with the goal of identifying the body. As in other cases, we have utilized two basic work strategies to effect positive identifications. First, there is the anthropological process, which consists of comparing the antemortem physical information given by the victims' families with the data gleaned from the exhumation and laboratory work. Unfortunately, the antemortem data from families is not always sufficient or decisive enough to provide a positive identification. Antemortem data from medical or dental records is reliable in most cases, but is often not consistently available.

Secondly, and simultaneous to the first comparison of physical data, there is the historic research, which traces individual fates through written sources, such as the archives of the CONADEP, judicial proceedings, death certificates, cemetery records, autopsy reports, and the archives of the Federal Police. Although we have begun to discern the manner by which individuals were imprisoned and transferred between sites, as explained above, these are among the most difficult hypotheses to establish with any certainty.

The lack of sufficient antemortem data, the complexity of the repression, similarities in the general biological profile of the victims, and insufficient access to DNA analysis, have all been factors contributing to the low numbers of positive identifications in Sector 134. At the time of writing, 17 individuals have been positively identified, by the use of historical and anthropological methods, and DNA testing.

CONCLUSIONS

Principally, it is of great importance to remember that the work presented in this chapter refers to what was accomplished long before anthropologists and archaeologists had started to take part as a matter of course in investigations connected with human rights violations. Therefore, technical problems arose during excavation procedures, and additionally within the laboratory analysis, which had to be dealt with by the application of specific and often novel solutions.

Furthermore, far from the habitual environment of academia, in which longer periods of time can be taken to study recovered remains and associated data, to formulate results, and where no pressure can be reasonably expected to be applied from surviving relatives to produce results rapidly, new strategies had to be developed pertaining to interactions with judges, prosecutors and lawyers, the media, and other players involved.

Additionally, owing to the close contact established with the witnesses and victim's relatives, members of the EAAF had to learn how to be respectful and sensitive to their desires, doubts and pain, whilst performing their scientific tasks thoroughly (Doretti and Fondebrider, 2004; Doretti and Fondebrider, 2001).

In conclusion, the investigation performed in Sector 134 of Avellaneda Cemetery, long before the period known as "forensic anthropology and human rights", has proved that conducting an exhaustive historical research into the identity of the victims, and circumstances in which they disappeared and were murdered, is bound to the archaeological recovery of their remains and their subsequent analysis. It also served to illustrate that technical challenges are just part of the problem, and that political, judicial and psychological issues have to be borne in mind before, during, and after such an investigation.

REFERENCES

Buikstra, J.E., and Ubelaker, D.H. (Eds.) (1994). *Standards for data collections from human skeletal remains.* Fayetteville: Arkansas Archaeological Survey Research.

DiMaio, V.J.M. (1985). *Gunshot wounds: Practical aspects of firearms, ballistics, and forensic techniques.* New York: Elsevier.

Doretti, M., and Fondebrider, L. (2001). Science and human rights: Truth, justice, reparation and reconciliation: A long way in third world countries. In *Archaeologies of the Contemporary Past*, Buchli, V., and Gavin, L. (Eds.). London: Routledge, pp. 138–144.

Doretti, M., and Fondebrider, L. (2004). Perspectives and recommendations from the field: Forensic anthropology and human rights in Argentina. *Proceedings of the 56th Academy of Forensic Sciences Meeting, Feb. 16–21, Dallas, Texas.* Annual Meeting of the American Academy of Forensic Sciences, Dallas.

Doretti, M., and Snow, C. (2003). Forensic anthropology and human rights: The Argentine experience. In *Hard evidence: Case studies in forensic anthropology*, Steadman, D.W. (Ed.). Upper Saddle River: Prentice Hall, pp. 290–310.

Ferllini Timms, R. (1993). *Principios de arqueología forense.* San José: Universidad Estatal a Distancia.

Fondebrider, L. (2004). *Uncovering evidence: The forensic sciences in human rights.* US: Project of the Center for Victims of Torture.

Fondebrider, L. (2005). Notas para una historia de la antropología forense en Latinoamérica. *ERES Arqueología/Bioantropología, 13*:127–136.

Fondebrider, L., and Mendonca, M.C. (2001). *Model protocol on the forensic investigation of death suspected to have been caused by a human rights violation.* Geneva: Office of the

United Nations High Commissioner for Human Rights.

France, D. L., Griffin, T.J., Swanburg, J.G., Lindemann, J.W., Davenport, G.C., Trammell, V., Travis, C.T., Kondratieff, B., Nelson, A., Castellano, K., Hopkins, D., and Adair, T. (1992). A multidisciplinary approach to the detection of clandestine graves. *J. Forensic Sciences, 37*(6):1445–1458.

Grauer, A.L. (Ed.) (1995). *Bodies of evidence: Reconstructing history through skeletal analysis.* New York: Wiley-Liss.

Haglund, W. (2001). Archaeology and forensic death investigations. *Historical Archaeology, 35*:26–34.

Haglund, W., Connor, M., and Scott, D. (2001). The archaeology of contemporary mass graves. *Historical Archaeology, 35*:57–69.

Haglund, W., and Sorg, M. (Eds.) (1997). *Forensic taphonomy: The postmortem fate of human remains.* Boca Raton: CRC Press.

Hunter, J., Brickley, M.B., Bourgeois, J., Bouts, W., Bourguignon, L., Hubrecht, F., DeWinne, J., Van Haaster, H., Hakbul, T., De Jong, H., Smits, L., Van Wijngaarden, L.H., Luschen, M. (2001). Forensic archaeology, forensic anthropology, and human rights in Europe. *Science and Justice, 4*:173–178.

Hunter, J.R., Roberts, C., and Martin, A. (1996). *Studies in crime: An introduction to forensic archaeology.* London: Batsford (Reprinted 1997, by Routledge: London).

Morse D., Duncan J., and Stoutamire, J. (Eds.) (1983). *Handbook of forensic archaeology and anthropology.* Tallahassee: Florida State University Foundation, Inc.

Rodríguez, J.V. (1994). *Introducción a la antropología forense: Análisis e interpretación de restos óseos humanos.* Colombia: Anaconda.

Sigler-Eisenberg, B. (1985). Forensic research: Expanding the concept of applied archaeology. *American Antiquity, 50*:650–655.

Skinner, M.F. (1987). Planning the archaeological recovery of evidence from recent mass graves. *Forensic Science International, 34*:267–287.

Skinner, M.F., Alempijevic, D., and Djuric-Srejic, M. (2003). Guidelines for international forensic bioarchaeology monitors of mass grave exhumations. *Forensic Science International, 134*:81–92.

Skinner, M.F., and Sterenberg, J. (2005). Turf wars: Authority and responsibility for the investigation of mass graves. *Forensic Science International, 151*:221–232.

Snow, C. (1984a). The investigation of the human remains of the 'disappeared' in Argentina. *American Journal of Medicine and Pathology, 5*:297–300.

Snow, C. (1984b). Forensic anthropology in the documentation of human rights abuses. *American Journal of Forensic Medicine and Pathology, 5*:297–299.

Snow, C., and Bihurriet, M.J. (1992). An epidemiology of homicide: Ningún nombre burials in the Province of Buenos Aires from 1970 to 1984. In *Human rights and statistics: Getting the record straight,* Jabine, T.B., and Claude, C.P. (Eds.). Philadelphia: University of Philadelphia Press, pp. 328–363.

Ubelaker, D.H. (1989). *Human skeletal remains: Excavation, analysis, interpretation.* Washington, D.C.: Taraxacum.

United Nations (1991). *Manual on the effective prevention and investigation of extra-legal, arbitrary and summary executions.* New York: Center for Social Development and Humanitarian Affairs.

Workshop of European Anthropologists (1980). Recommendations for age and sex diagnoses. *Journal of Human Evolution, 9*:517–549.

Chapter 10

HAPLESS IN AFGHANISTAN:
FORENSIC ARCHAEOLOGY IN
A POLITICAL MAELSTROM

MARK SKINNER

INTRODUCTION

This is a personal account of my experiences as an ingénue forensic archaeologist in Afghanistan in 1997. I was seconded by
Physicians for Human Rights (PHR) to the UN High Commissioner
for Human Rights to investigate allegations of mass graves purported
to contain remains of some 1,200 Taliban prisoners recently executed
by the Northern Alliance forces. Our mission was to seek evidence of
mass graves, their number, the approximate number of victims, and
their manner and cause of death. In reality, the team was able to determine with confidence only that a great many human remains existed on the surface at some of these sites; that in the same area there
existed ballistic evidence in abundance, that some individuals were
bound, and that the deaths had probably occurred that year. The
forensic meaning of the evidence was uncertain, pending proper investigation; particularly, one could not assume that buried evidence
existed at all, or would provide the same inferences as did that on the
surface.

My report, and subsequent advocacy of proper forensic investigation
of selected sites was obviated by political developments. In conclusion,
only a combination of in-depth forensic investigation, supported by sustained political will, can effectively deal with mass killings in conflict
areas.

THE SETTING

I was in Afghanistan, in the rain shadow of the near-desert north of the Hindu Kush Mountains. It was December, 1997. I was there on behalf of Physicians for Human Rights to assist the UN's Special Rapporteur for Afghanistan. Our mission was to investigate alleged mass graves said to contain the remains of some 1,200 missing Taliban fighters taken prisoner by an alliance of northern warlords. It was my first experience as a forensic anthropologist working internationally. I looked at a row of mummified feet sticking out of the sand. I watched a large black beetle negotiate an exposure-whitened femur. A cartridge case, examined and discarded by one of us, had rolled down a sandy slope, creating an artful curve in the sand. I thought "I can handle this. It's like the short-grass cattle country of Southern Alberta where I grew up – only worse."

HISTORICAL-POLITICAL BACKGROUND

Afghanistan has always been strategically important; forming, historically, a buffer between British dominated India/Pakistan in the south and Russia to the north who wanted access to a warm water port and an oil pipeline. Afghanistan's involvement in the opium trade combined with its natural gas resources and geopolitical setting attracted international influences in the so-called Petrodollar era; notably Islamic Iran and Communist USSR who competed for control of the region. During the Cold War era, financial support was provided from various countries for revolutionary elites. Soviet occupation occurred in 1980, ostensibly for six months. By 1985, natural gas sales to USSR accounted for 40 percent of the annual income in Afghanistan. In turn, huge arms sales were made to President Najibullah to the tune of 3–4 billion dollars per year. At the same time, the Mujahadin (Islamic resistance fighters) received 1 billion dollars from U.S. and Saudi Arabia; most military aid was in personal weapons (machine guns), shipped through Pakistan and not American made but controlled by the Central Intelligence Agency (CIA). There was considerable resistance within Afghanistan to foreign influence-especially Soviet. In 1985, Mikhail Gorbachev came to power and started to grapple with the problem of Afghanistan which he called his "bleeding wound." Of about 16 million citizens, over one million Afghanis had been killed in anti-soviet fighting, 2–3 million more had been internally displaced and

5 million had left the country. In 1991, Gorbachev announced the dissolution of the USSR, stopped shipping arms to Afghanistan and withdrew Soviet forces. Ten years of soviet occupation were followed by 10 years of civil war. An entire generation has grown up there with no formal education and no basic social infrastructure (Rubin, 1996).

The society has been described as tribal, feudal and feuding but this is simplistic and dismissive; the invasion and withdrawal of Soviet occupation forces created a chaotic nation riven by civil war with combatants armed from international sources with land mines and Kelashnikov rifles, and so the inhabitants turned to Islamic fundamentalism to find a means of restoring order. At the time of our investigation in late 1997, the civil war was being fought between northern and southern forces. The Northern Alliance was an unstable amalgam of five generals (warlords) formerly dominated by General Abdul Malik, but since ousted by General Abdul Rashid Dostum with a base in Mazar I Sharif, where he looked after the vital natural gas resources and roads to the north. The southern forces were called the Taliban, students of Islamic religion educated in Pakistan which relies on the Shari'a-Islamic law and traditional tribal justice since there was no functioning judicial system. They are Sunni Muslim unified by adherence to an extreme form of Islamic fundamentalism. Non-Taliban forces, with whom they are fighting, are mostly Shi'a. The west is very critical of the Taliban treatment of women who are usually required to wear a Burqa and are denied basic rights of education and health care (Constable, 1999). Male control of women is called pardah which involves the segregation and seclusion of women. Veiling is termed chadri. However, it is clear that the Taliban's fundamentalism was generating a stable, unified political and military force that was winning the civil war in Afghanistan. Between 1997, the time of our investigation, and 1999 the land area controlled by the Taliban increased from 65 percent to 95 percent. On October 7, 2001 Afghanistan was invaded by American forces responding to the September 11, 2001 attacks on the World Trade Centre and Pentagon on the grounds that Afghanistan harboured terrorist agents of Al Qaeda.

THE POLITICAL SITUATION IN 1997

In May, 1997 there was a major battle in the city of Shiberghan in northern Afghanistan west of Mazar (Fig. 10-1). There were many

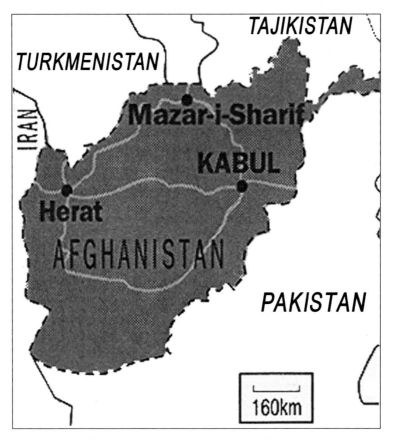

Figure 10-1. Afghanistan: Shiberghan, the base of operations, is located just west of Mazar.

deaths. In addition, approximately 1,600 Taliban soldiers were captured. In mid-June allegedly 100 soldiers at a time were taken from the prison and executed. One thousand two hundred prisoners were missing. In late 1997, General Dostum invited the United Nations High Commissioner for Human Rights (UNHCHR) to Afghanistan to view five alleged mass graves said to contain the missing soldiers. The perpetrators were said to be northern forces under the control of General Malik. It was clear that General Dostum's political ambition was to consolidate his leadership over the northern forces, even though it showed his enemy the Taliban as victims rather than aggressors. In a letter to the High Commissioner for Human Rights dated 10 December, 1997 addressing the issue of missing Taliban prisoners, General Malik characterized General Dostum as follows:

General Dostum whose ancestors had cooperated with the Bolsheviks in the fall of Bokharu . . . became a member of the Soviet Intelligence; i.e., the KGB and later was sent to the former Soviet Union to earn a higher education in the field. [] After the withdrawal of the Red Army from Afghanistan in 1989, he was responsible for conducting criminal acts and continuing wars waged by the Communist regime against the innocent people of Afghanistan.

Now, in order to cover the crimes he has committed over the last 18 years and because of his personal enmity against myself and the Islamic State of Afghanistan, General Dostum is once again under the order of the Pakistani military intelligence attempting to launch widespread publicity campaign called "Discovery of mass Taliban graves." The killings in fact may have been the total number in the battles of Mazar-I-Sharif, Faryab, Sheberghan and elsewhere in the north. On the one hand, he wants to politically discredit me and the Islamic State of Afghanistan and on the other, cover his two-decade long criminal acts.

As a westerner, I had been inculcated with the view that the Taliban were the "bad guys." As a forensic scientist, I was expected to be politically neutral. As a member of a UN Team hosted by General Dostum, I was expected to be, if nothing else, polite. As a Canadian, I think it is fair to say, I was expected to be nice.

FORENSIC INVOLVEMENT

The assistance of a forensic anthropologist was requested from Physicians for Human Rights by the UNHCHR to participate with Prof. Choong-Hyun Paik, Special Rapporteur on Human Rights for Afghanistan, to provide a preliminary assessment of reports of mass graves in northern Afghanistan (Fig. 10-2). The graves were purported to contain bodies of executed Taliban prisoners – an apparent abuse of human rights. It was generally acknowledged that ours was a preliminary effort, designed to plan further investigations if warranted by the evidence. Our mandate was:

- to seek evidence of mass graves
- to find the number of such graves in designated areas
- to find the approximate number of individuals involved
- to determine the manner and cause of death

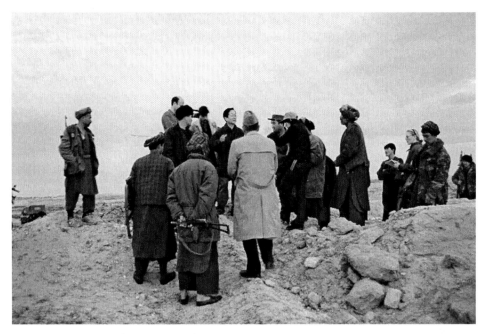

Figure 10-2. Dr. Paik (facing camera), Special Rapporteur on Human Rights to Afghanistan, with team.

Dec. 8th, 1997 – in Marriott Hotel in Islamabad – it's bucketing down outside-not what I expected. I landed not quite 24 hours ago and have spent most of that time dozing and trying to deal with this god awful cold. I've had no luck contacting my UN person here; have learned the home phone number is wrong. The trucks and taxis here are metal gypsy wagons – swooping tops and vivid garish colours and metal disks on chains by the hundred – very odd; rode with an African-Indian lady from British Embassy with a sister in Calgary who lamented the corruption in Pakistan and India. Yellow pages disproportionately full of ads for surgical instruments and hunting knives.

Dec. 9th – it's 3:40 AM and I've woken up. Managed a couple of good hours sleep. Have planned all day; last night I met the UN Human Rights Team consisting of Dr. Paik (a Korean lawyer); Darka Topali, his assistant, and Irene Abrahamian, an interpreter. They were very tired and hungry but let me accompany them to their late dinner. We watched a video made by supporters of General Dostum who desires the exhumation of allegedly Taliban graves to discredit his political opponent – one Malik, I believe. Bodies are very superficial; very disturbed. Looks like mummification and skeletonization combined. I've worked out a strategy to sample this bizarre universe. Learned from video that 10" spikes won't do – shifting sands. Tomorrow (today) will be hectic trying to find supplies I need but I think I'll have a driver at my disposal.

Dec. 10th – Int'l Human Rights day; how apropos. On UN plane to Shiberghan with 3 UN personnel, Prof. Paik and BBC reporter Alan Johnson. Have explained my strategy and no one has objected. My plans and schedule take priority but I anticipate delays. I hope to be on site by 2 PM. I have topo maps and bamboo stakes, so soon it'll be entirely up to me.

When we first got to site with General Dostum there were close to 100 soldiers with an alarming number of Kelashnikovs and shovels. They were ready to dig up the whole area. I asked for General Dostum to confirm that any diggers were to be commanded by me.

The full team was shown six areas designated as follows:

1. *The Dump Site* – a bone strewn mound of earth, 3 km west of Shiberghan, at a village garbage disposal area (Fig. 10-3).

2. *The Shiberghan Desert Site* – scattered concentrations of human bones lying on the surface and clearly scavenged by animals, spread over a kilometer or more in the desert immediately west of the previously-mentioned site (Fig. 10-4).

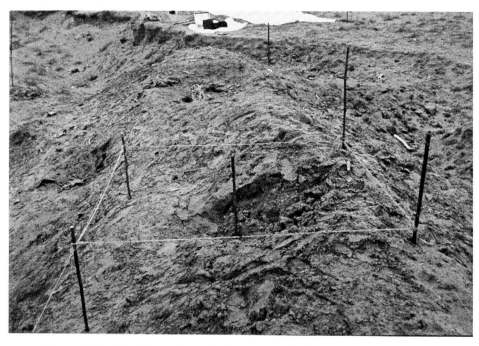

Figure 10-3. The Dump Site with 2 metre unit laid out prior to excavation.

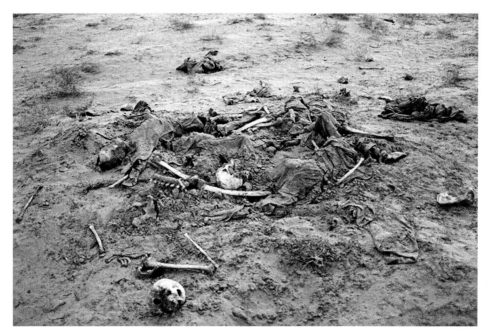

Figure 10-4. The Shiberghan Desert Site.

3. *The Nine Wells Site* – a group of nine water wells in the rolling dunes 19 km west of Shiberghan alleged to contain the remains of anywhere between 400 to 1600 unlawfully executed prisoners forced down the wells at gunpoint; with additional use of a grenade and bulldozer to obliterate the evidence (Fig. 10-5).

4. *Hairatan Highway Desert Site* – scattered concentrations of fairly intact bodies behind dunes to west of highway roughly mid-way between Mazar-I-Sharif and Hairatan (Fig. 10-6).

5. *The Ridge Site* – a row of quite intact bodies on both sides of a wide ridge slightly north of the previous site on the east side of the highway (Fig. 10-7 and 10-8).

6. *Two villages* – (Qizilabad, Sheikhabad) near Mazar at which locals have given traditional burials to civilians allegedly tortured and killed by Taliban soldiers.

5:45 PM – I just noticed my fridge has bullet holes in it. Funny I kept asking myself why my room smelled like dead sheep. Maybe someone copped it in here. Bullets came through window – one passing through a wall, door and into bathroom. 10:15 as I go to bed I've found a bullet hole above my bed frame.

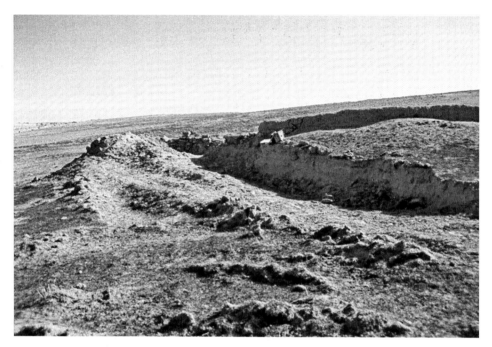

Figure 10-5. The Nine Wells Site: bulldozed well.

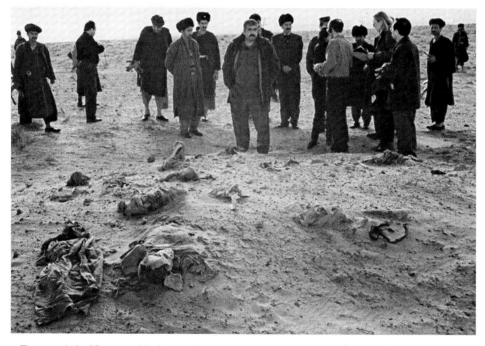

Figure 10-6. Hairatan Highway Desert Site: General Dostum (with hands in pockets).

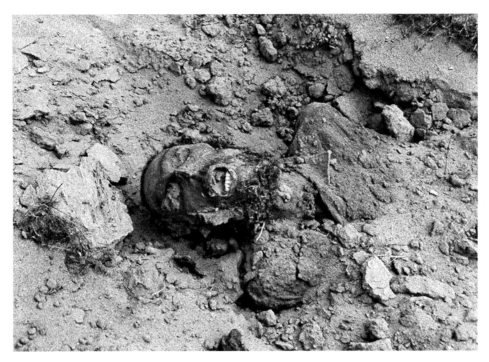

Figure 10-7. The Ridge Site: body exposed by Dostum's soldiers; arms are pinioned.

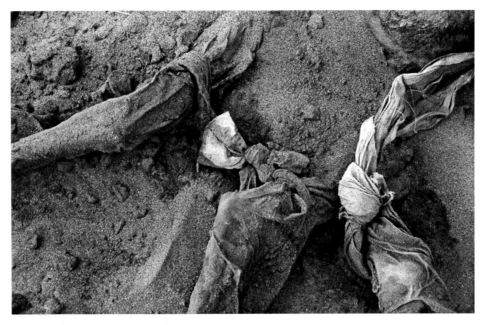

Figure 10-8. Pinioned elbows.

Thurs. Dec. 11th – my interpreter is Mr. Gurd. 72 years old – he was sleeping when required to come to Dostum's Guest House. No plugs in sink or bath, so I used drinking glasses as plugs.

I have a particularly vivid memory of being asked to be present during the statement of an informant at General Dostum's guest house where we were staying. We were taken to a very large room dominated at one end by the largest TV screen I have ever seen, but non-functioning due to a bullet hole in one corner. At the other end, was an equally imposing chair in which Dostum sat. Our team was grouped around in plush chairs and furnished with cups of tea. A turbaned man was led in. He knelt directly in front of Dostum, bowed, and recounted his tale of assisting with the execution of Taliban prisoners on orders of General Malik, who had recently vacated the area. As I looked at Dostum, the phrase "oriental potentate" came to mind. Dostum was notorious for his actions; for example, he is alleged to have disciplined one of his soldiers by tying him between two tanks, and ordering them to drive in opposite directions. We asked why this perpetrator was not imprisoned. Dostum replied through his interpreter that the informant was not going anywhere. Indeed, the perpetrators were Northern Alliance soldiers, who now worked for Dostum.

Well, it's now evening; day was totally different than expected; this morning was eating my three eggs and biscuits with honey when I was told General Dostum was expecting me also to accompany UN team to Hairatan. I was told to bring my stuff to dig up a body-sounded ominous; but I grabbed my stuff and ran. Dressed totally wrong-all in my super-insulating black thermal underwear and shirt and overalls-only to sit three abreast in back seat of land cruiser all day. We went to three sites and two villages. Trip back very stupefying cause of heat in truck. Our morning's armed guard included several soldiers with rocket launchers, the lot had dwindled by evening to a single solider with a Kelashnikov who sat behind my head. Had a nice meal with UN staff; I will miss them. My plane lands on Tues at 2 PM so I'll have 3 full days to work at site.

Fri. Dec. 12th – this AM off to see 3 water wells; depth varied from 30–60' [10–20 m] and by sound of dropped rock very deep water at bottom. The wells are brick-lined at top 8' [2 m]; although I think first well was brick-lined whole way to 30'. But "filled-in" wells supposed to be like the very deep ones. Well diameter is quite narrow maybe 1.2 m.; opens wide to max. 2 m at various levels. Sides look stable. Hard sandstone-packed earth or something – so not likely to slump as bodies removed (unless weakened by grenade); idea of excavating from side seems much less feasible now.

DECISION TIME

The UN team had spent a couple of days visiting sites and being briefed by General Dostum. We accepted most of what we were told although, of course, I did not know exactly what Professor Paik would advise the UNHCHR. I was aware that the UN Team would provide a public statement that we had been shown several mass graves and that these contained, as alleged by Dostum, Taliban prisoners improperly taken out and executed. I felt uneasy about my own abilities to deal with mass graves to any degree as well as the exact nature of the varied sites we had seen. So I asked permission from the General as well as the UN Team to stay behind to undertake an actual excavation. I rejected the surface execution sites as their contents were pretty obvious and had been rather badly impacted by scavengers and Dostum's soldiers. Similarly, I decided not to attempt to excavate any portion of the Ridge Site as it was forensically very important – given the evidence of ligatures and ballistics. Also the "Nine Wells Site" was far too logistically challenging for me to tackle by myself. The "Dump Site" was selected for test excavation because the earth mound was reported to have been created by local villagers over the decaying bodies soon after they appeared and because of accessibility from a base at General Dostum's Guest House in Shiberghan. My understanding of this site was that it contained executed Taliban prisoners whose bodies had been gathered up by locals. I worked alone using the most basic supplies gathered earlier by me en route through Islamabad. I had no GPS (Global Positioning System), or surveying equipment. I did have a measuring tape, trowel, and compass.

Forensic archaeology is a distinct suite of skills very rarely possessed by anthropologists, particularly those from North America who use the terms forensic archaeology and anthropology interchangeably. In my opinion, forensic archaeology has emerged as a distinct discipline particularly due to the efforts of British and Australian practitioners (Wright et al., 2005). While in Afghanistan I practiced both specialties and threw in a dash of forensic pathology. The disquieting suspicion of "dabbling" has led subsequently to our advocating more thoughtful allocation of forensic expertise at mass graves (Skinner and Sterenberg, 2005).

The Dump Site

Spatial Control

The Dump Site was an elongated mound of earth, ca. 18 m long by 3–4 m wide by 1–2 m deep, oriented east-west within a complex of wind erosion gullies adjacent to a traditional garbage dump. Numerous bones and fragments of clothing were scattered on the mound and nearby areas. A 2 m wide swath through the centre of the long axis of the mound was laid out with string and bamboo poles. This swath was divided into nine-two metre units, of which Unit 0–2 mN and 6–8 mE were selected for excavation, as they were roughly in the centre and, apart from slumpage, appeared undisturbed (Fig. 10-3). This amounted to roughly 12 percent of the mounded earth judged likely to contain evidence.

Time Table

Three and a half days were allotted for processing the selected unit:
  I. First half-day (Friday, Dec. 12, 1997) – grid control and removal of ca. 50 cm overburden.
  II. First full day (Dec. 13) – excavation to expose bodies.
  III. Second full day (Dec. 14) – excavation to remove all bodies to sterile- depth of ca. 60–90 cm.
  IV. Third full day (Dec. 15) – postmortem examination of ten recovered partial or complete bodies; reburial.

At noon after farewell meeting with General Dostum at which we were all presented with very nice rugs, the UN team went back to Islamabad. We had to wait a very long two hours before Alan Johnston badgered Mr. Usman into taking us into field. His son, I think, Forzel became my assistant. Excavated first NW quadrant to 60 cm below *datum* at SW corner; first subsurface evidence in SW quadrant at 60 cm depth; could be cloth or hair. Forzel found this.

He became more and more upset as we began to get close to what we strongly suspected would be bodies. I'm pretty sure that my corner posts went into bodies; but as I think about it maybe not. Indeed the body we eventually encountered may be lying on ground surface. All I've uncovered so far, in SW quadrant is front teeth and nose. In SE quadrant, covering fill contained 1 vertebra and 2 unfired bullets – the latter at about 50 cm depth – 10 cm above body in adjacent square. Why are bullets not fired? Alan does a lot of filming and I did a small blurb on intent; I suppose it'll be on BBC Radio International tonight.

The discovery of unspent cartridges was my first hint, unperceived at the time, that these remains were not those of executed prisoners. I knew it did not make sense. The vexed question of "association" between the remains and the ballistic evidence began to niggle at my mind. Also, why were there isolated bones in the grave fill?-something else that did not make sense.

Sat. Dec. 13th – 7:20 still no breakfast and not in field. I've been planning autopsy methods but today may be spent entirely on exposing bodies. Have just read the UN document containing Taliban proclamation on acceptable women's behavior – they can only work as nurses and must not be noisy with their feet. The religious police beat offending women and stop men to inspect their private parts to see if they've been shaved. It's not simply gender discrimination, but zealotry directed against all citizenry.

Spent all day exposing at least 4 bodies. Smell got to me around 2 PM – so last three hours were horrendous. I think cause my stomach was empty. Once Alan Johnson told me to look up and there on the near horizon were 3 donkeys and 2 camels – a perfect Christmas scene. Also saw an eagle. The bodies have a lot of soft tissue in nether regions. I was able to expose a natural bank surface against which two of the bodies are tightly pressed. But the whole body mass is on quite a slope. The wealth of clothing is a bugger; esp. as I don't understand it. It's flowing baggy pants, top, patu and maybe turban. One brand name has shown up. Also there's enigmatic thick plastic folded against one tibia. It's only 8 o'clock but I'm knackered; I've washed my boots and overalls. Having Alan here is an absolute god send.

Around this time, I realized that my unfamiliarity with local material culture and burial customs was detrimental to good forensic archaeology. Indeed, I needed a local cultural anthropologist to advise me (Fig. 10-9).

Sun. Dec. 14th – It's now 6:45 AM and I've been awake since 4. No electricity till 5. I've spent the time reading about Afghanistan's fractured politics and cutting body numbers out of plastic water bottles. The numbers are for re-interment in case anyone wants to dig them up again – not a strong possibility. I've rubbed underarm deodorant on my face mask (outside) to see if this will make the smell less offensive. Darka took the Chanel #5 away with her.

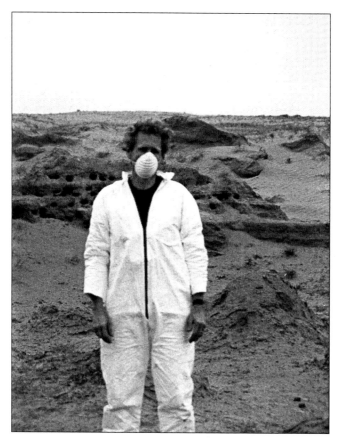

Figure 10-9. The author.

The plan today is to sketch body position, photograph under better light, then lift and autopsy. Yesterday, I had to open up the North face of the pit due to slumpage of the unconsolidated earth; this was a blessing in disguise as it made access to the bodies a lot easier. The entire floor of the pit is covered with clothing draped over bones. Nowhere to stand. Have to bend over and reach all the time which is very tiring.

Site Security

Site security which Mr. Gurd helped me arrange was 2 armed guards at a time throughout the night. I sure hope they kept the dogs away cause the first night a dog dug up some scalp hair. When we arrived at the site yesterday we were not allowed near. Alan thought they might be checking for mines planted in the night presumably in the pit. Horrid thought.

There was some shooting and chasing but it did not seem to be a big deal so we simply started work.

On the evening of Dec. 12, 1997 a dog dug up some scalp hair in the southeast 1m quadrant. Consequently, on the following evening after complete exposure of the uppermost five bodies in preparation for photography, armed guards were posted, two at a time. This was ineffectual; during the night dogs seriously damaged the site pulling out the *datum* pole, pit strings and collapsing some earth onto the remains. Only one bone was pulled out and chewed. The dogs in Afghanistan were very scary; their ears and tails were docked by shepherds so that when they fought they wouldn't bleed so much.

I was very upset that the guards had not protected the site during the night. My careful exposure of the remains and brushing the sand away for photography the next day was wasted time. I made it clear that I was unhappy with the guards and did not speak to anyone for about three hours while I worked. Eventually, the BBC reporter told me the disturbing tale that once, when another investigative reporter writing a story on Dostum's activities in the North lost a camera to a thief and complained about it, the thief was shot on the spot. That my guards were replaced left me with a disquieting uncertainty about their fate.

Sun. Dec. 14th cont. – It's now 8:30 PM and I've communed with the dead all day. 10 in the pit every which way. Liquefying flesh with maggots and coffin flies very active. Apparently all summer clothes. Most show bullet wounds to bone and 1 shows a frame for fractured tibia while another has bandages. These are crudest of field palliatives. Several with bullets in flesh; turned green while bullets are silver. These were copper-jacketed I think.

My gear (esp. boots) really smelled. I had put underarm on my face mask; worked like a damn. Dogs had wrecked my picture perfect pit. The guard was punished. God I hope the guards look after all 10 discrete individuals which are now out of pit and very vulnerable.

Around this time, I began to encounter physical evidence of medical treatment of severe battle wounds. That, combined, with unspent cartridges in pockets of one individual got me thinking that these individuals could hardly be considered prisoners.

Mon. Dec. 15th – evening – did 10 autopsies today; learned a lot. Everything supports conclusion that these are grievously-wounded and dead combatants taken to the dump and dumped. Their clothes are Taliban as are the beards apparently. Two individuals had bandages and/or splints but very simple which suggests field medical treatment; not necessarily hospital. Re: bullets from #8's body – it was pointing into body so I concluded shot from front but the bullet's base is badly distorted; could it have tumbled? Mr. Gurd helped me interpret clothing. I collected no insect evidence-the flies had flown (they were in dirt, in bodies but still myriad maggots esp. in wet areas). Alan did a radio interview and then a video so I'll be on BBC TV next week I guess. I stated that a neutral team of international investigators should look at well area and ridge near Ayratan [Hairatan]. I hope P.H.R. and UN don't mind my giving interview. I did say that the area I had investigated did *not* contain non-combatants; but rather those wounded and killed in battle. Nothing about the trauma suggests deliberate execution. One thing bothers me; in 2 individuals 3 fibulae are shot away in same place but missed tibiae. How can this happen to a single individual? Looks almost like some kind of knee-capping. I reburied each individual in wrapped plastic with plastic body number in a spot 17 metres north and very slightly east of my primary *datum*. The workers treated it like a proper grave. Mr. Gurd who is also a mullah advised me to place the heads to the north which I did. I gave my knife and some toffee to the guard who helped me wrap the bodies. I won't be leaving here tomorrow – technical problem with plane but Alan says we are flying right into Hindu Kush and it's beautiful.

I am still puzzled by the bilateral fibular head fractures. They are uncommon and are usually caused by a direct blow or a varus stress on the knee due to forceful contraction of the biceps femoris during an epileptic seizure.

The following is an extract from my report to the UN (Skinner, 1998).

Findings at the Dump Site

A. **Site Formation and Depth Below Surface:** An elderly shepherd discovered bodies at a dump located just west of the junction of the main highway leading west out of Shiberghan and a paved north-south highway three km. west of the centre of Shiberghan. Persons unknown rolled the bodies over a roughly 2 m high bank. Because of the smell, locals dug dirt over the bodies to a depth of about 20 cm above highest ground level.

Excavation revealed a hidden bank over which the bodies had been tumbled; the most upslope bodies being barely below the original ground surface. The villagers had dug a ditch about 1 metre in from the bank's edge to generate the earth to cover the bodies. The bank slopes about 50 cm over the 2 metre extent revealed by excavation. At no place were the remains more than two bodies deep. The maximum earth cover over the bodies was about 70 cm. The tangled loose, flowing clothing and blankets made extrication of individual bodies difficult (Fig. 10-10).

B. **Time of Death:** The interpreter explained that the clothing of all bodies was summer wear. No vegetation had commenced regrowth on the mound's surface. At depth, in moist areas under the bodies, numerous insect larvae were encountered as well as many adult flies. The bodies were more fleshed than skeletonized except where no cloth protected the remains; hence most heads were basically skulls with adherent scalp and facial hair. The habitat is desertic. Based on these considerations, death is reconstructed to have occurred 3–9 months prior to excavation; i.e., between April and September, 1997. The investigators had been told that many Taliban were killed or captured in May, 1997.

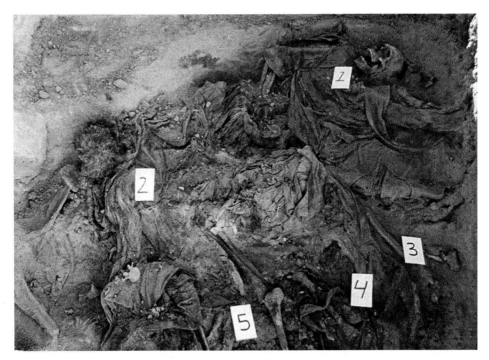

Figure 10-10. The Dump Site: upper layer of bodies.

C. **Number of Bodies:** The more or less complete remains of 10 individuals were recovered from a 4 sq. metre area excavated to sterile. This represents roughly 12 percent of the total mound (edges being subtracted); i.e., a total of 83 bodies are estimated to be at the Dump Site. According to the shepherd who found the bodies, there were 10 in 10 rows – about 100. The difference in the two estimates is negligible.

D. **Description of Individuals:** This is summarized in Table 10-1, so comments are restricted to noteworthy observations.

TABLE 10-1. RESULTS OF EXAMINATION OF TEN YOUNG MALES

Body	Preservation	Trauma	Clothing	Artifacts	Comment
1	whole skeleton feet fleshed	cervical 6 fractured	blue waistcoat shirt loose trousers beaded tassle	unspent cartridge string	bearded
2	whole body much flesh/skin	none	square shawl shirt undershirt trousers	knotted plastic ring ca. 3 cm dia.	two loops in ring
3	pelvis and legs fleshed	lt. fibula fractured	trousers	none	upper body absent
4	fleshed legs only no hips	grooved lt. femur head	trousers	plastic pouch with objects	skeletally full adult
5	legs only little flesh	none	none	none	
6	whole body skeletonized fleshy feet brain matter	fractures of lt. fibula rt. fibula	shirt trousers	2 blankets 3 bandages 'sock' plastic ring amulet	received treatment for wounds
7	whole body long beard mostly fleshed	frac. vertebra fractured rib frac. lt. femur fract rt. femur frac. rt. tibia	waistcoat trousers	"patu" shawl beaded tassle arm amulet 19 boxed cartridges splint	Afghani money splinted leg 1 steel bullet
8	whole body individual except lo. legs fleshed	shattered rt. scapula bullet groove in femur	shirt waistcoat trousers	one bullet	youngest *(cont'd.)*

TABLE 10-1. RESULTS OF EXAMINATION OF TEN YOUNG MALES *(Cont'd.)*

Body	Preservation	Trauma	Clothing	Artifacts	Comment
9	head and left arm; hand fleshed	frac. distal lt. ulna massive facial fractures	none	none	heavily bearded dentally full adult
10	upper body much soft tissue	skull base bullet wound	blanket shirt	cigarettes and matches	

Sex was determined primarily from the pubic bone or pelvis; as well as facial hair. All individuals were male. Age indicators included third molar eruption, basilar suture fusion, sternal epiphysis fusion, pubic symphyseal appearance and epiphyseal fusion for limb bones. All individuals were subadults or young adults. Clothing ethnicity was tentatively identified by the interpreter.

Body Number One: Uppermost on the bank, this individual was represented by a complete body which was largely skeletonized except for the feet and some scalp hair; muscle shreds existed here and there. He was face-up. Both the waistcoat (brand Prince) and shirt have an apparent bullet hole angling upwards from behind; the bullet entered the neck completely detaching the neural arch of the sixth cervical vertebra. Shirt said to be "Badgis" while beaded tassle "maybe Herat."

Body Number Two: Lying somewhat beneath Body Numbers One and Five and covered with much clothing, this individual was largely fleshed which may explain my failure to observe skeletal trauma; bones could be pulled from fleshy lumps. He was face-down. The undershirt was brand Erika. The shawl ("towel") was described as "Herat or Kandahar." The trousers' beaded tassle was identified as "Herat." The two-looped small plastic ring is enigmatic (but there is a traditional practice of binding big toes together on a corpse)(Dupree, 1997). This artifact could be associated with the legs of Individual Number Five.

Body Number Three: This young adult was one of the oldest individuals. Only the hips and legs were present, lying ventral surface down. From the orientation of the legs in the pit the trunk should have been present. Much flesh was preserved, albeit dried, on the buttocks and knees; feet preserved with dissociable bones. Only the proximal 3 cm of the fractured left fibula was present; whereabouts of rest of fibular shaft not determined.

Body Number Four: This adult was represented by legs only; the rest of the body extended north beyond the excavated area. He was lying face-up. The left femoral head had a vertically-oriented groove, ca. 2 mm deep, 2 mm wide and 15 mm long on anterior surface. It was sand-filled. Its cause is unknown. A plastic pouch roughly 15 cm × 12 cm was lying against the left tibia at mid-shaft. It could easily be associated with a different individual. The contents of the pouch are as follows (Fig. 10-11):

- one digital watch (luxury quartz)-detached back with adherent cellotape
- one safety razor (sans blade) in three parts
- one brown, four-holed button (15 mm diameter)
- one roll of fine copper wire (ca. 50 cm long)
- one plastic electric cord gripper (missing one screw)
- one orange rectangular plastic button (cf. "Exacto" knife advance button)
- five machine screws (ca. 10 mm long): 3 flathead, 2 roundhead
- one tied black rubber band (rectangular in cross-section); cut from inner tube?

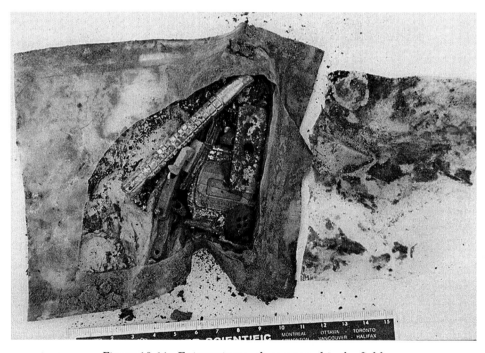

Figure 10-11. Enigmatic pouch as opened in the field.

- one 25 value coin (requires cleaning) with Arabic writing
- two dissimilar shaped, bent metal pieces; cf. electrical contacts for battery.

It has been suggested some of the contents (e.g., loop of wire) were consistent with material required to create a "booby trap"; the coin could be used as a screwdriver for the transit plug of an anti-personnel grenade. The machine screws are like those on the sight of a hand-held rocket launcher. Then again, the objects may be functionally unconnected.

Body Number Five: This individual is back-lying. He is represented only by legs with the rest of the body located to the north and outside of the excavated area. Little flesh was preserved. The plastic pouch (Body Number 4) may be from this body; or neither.

Body Number Six: This individual had several fractures as well as numerous artifacts. He was face down, roughly in the centre of the unit, apparently wrapped in two blankets. He had received medical or first-aid attention.

The right humerus was badly fractured over several centimetres of shaft near the head and extending to shaft one-third. Both fibulae were damaged in symmetrical locations. The left fibula is lacking the anterior half of the fibular head while the right fibular shaft was broken through just distal to the head. The tibiae were unaffected. The symmetrical nature of the fibular damage combined with unaffected tibiae is baffling. It probably reflects, not firearms injury, but sudden trauma to both legs planted on the ground.

Green strips of cloth, ca. 10 cm wide, were wound around the humerus and right fibula. That on the humerus was tied with a string (Fig. 10-12). It is assumed that the three bandages were associated with the three fractured limbs. In addition, a green tube "sock," which appears medical, was extricated from the mass of blankets and clothing. It could be associated with any of the injured limbs.

A circle of doubly-knotted plastic, roughly 20 cm in diameter, created from two tied pieces of plastic of unequal length was stuck to the face and encircled the head (Fig. 10-13). It was too big to be a blindfold or bandana. It appears to have functioned most likely as an arm sling for the damaged right arm; but this is speculative.

A cloth pillow amulet held with a cord around the neck was found under the chin. It is very similar to that found with Body Number Seven.

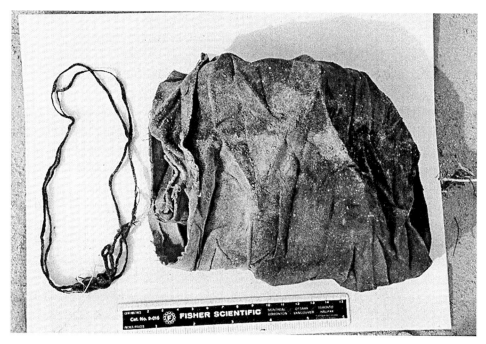

Figure 10-12. Field bandage from right humerus.

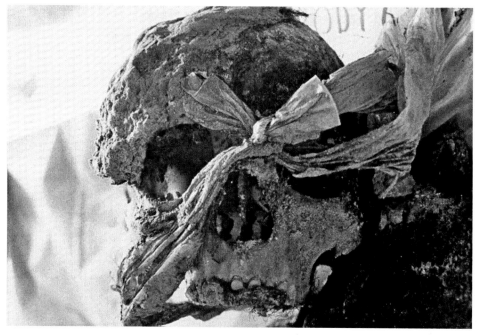

Figure 10-13. Plastic ring encircling head as observed in the field; a displaced sling.

Body Number Seven: The bones of this face-lying individual, also located in the approximate centre of the unit somewhat underneath and to the west of Body Number Six, still possessed fleshy remnants. He was fully clothed with a beaded tassle on his trouser belt which suggested a "Herat or Kandahar" origin. His waistcoat contained 110 Afghani in two paper notes as well as a disintegrating box containing 19 unspent cartridges (Kelashnikov rimless cartridges, 7.62 mm × 39 mm) plus, surprisingly, one spent bullet (sans copper gilding) of the same calibre. Around one humerus was the cord of a soft pillow amulet (an asymmetrical diamond shape) which, according to the interpreter, would probably contain a passage from the Koran.

Despite the remnant flesh, four fractures were observed: one lower thoracic vertebra was sheared in two (half not observed); one rib was broken through about 5 cm from vertebral end; the left femur was shattered into at least four pieces at about shaft one-third; and the right tibia was shattered, distally, at shaft two-thirds. The latter element was protected by a plastic-coated wire basket splint which cradled the back of the leg and supported the foot with an angled brace (Fig. 10-14). The splint was held to the lower leg by a gauze strip wrapping. The fibula

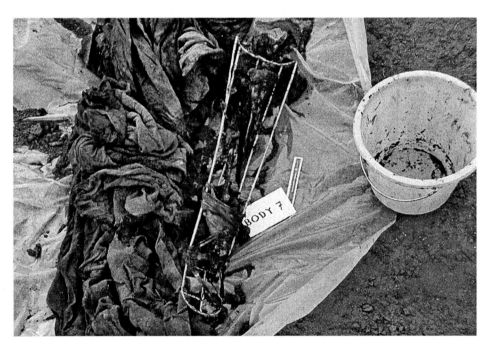

Figure 10-14. Field splint for shattered right leg.

was undamaged. Clearly this individual had received some sort of medical or first aid attention despite grievous, multiple wounds.

Body Number Eight: This individual, lying face down in the north half of the unit, deep to the legs of Bodies Three, Four and Five, was an older teenager; the distal femoral epiphysis was unfused at all. His clothing was unremarkable. He had been shot at least twice. The infraspinous region of the right scapula was badly shattered, with copper salts staining of the clavicle and humerus suggesting entry of the bullet from behind without it exiting the body. This bullet not recovered. The left femoral head was deeply grooved laterally and a steel bullet was found between it and the greater trochanter where it had stained the flesh a vivid green. The bullet's point suggested entry from in front and slightly to the victim's left side; although the bullet's base was slightly distorted. This bullet was retained. It is of the same calibre as noted above.

Body Number Nine: This face-up body extended largely out of the excavated area in the extreme northwest quadrant; hence, only the head and left arm were recovered. The face was massively fractured (both jaws in three pieces, frontal and right cheek bone fractured). There was no evidence of firearm injuries. The ulna was broken through at the wrist in the styloid region.

Body Number Ten: This face-lying individual's body extended mostly out of the west side of the excavated area; the recovered upper body had a lot of soft tissue holding the ribs together. The head was covered over with a blanket which helped preserve the scalp tissue and beard hair. There was severe trauma to the skull base. The presence of green staining on the left mastoid as well as the patterning of fractured bone suggested bullet entry on a horizontal plane in the right rear occipital, angling forward through the condyle/foramen magnum area to the other side. Presumably the bullet had not fully exited but it was not recovered.

E. **Summary of Evidence from Dump Site and Recommendations:** Remains of ten individuals, from an estimated total of 83, were excavated from an earthern mound. The state of decomposition, clothing and lack of plant regrowth suggests death in the summer, 1997. Several individuals had received sufficiently severe wounds as to suggest immediate death and yet two individuals had bandages or a splint to fractured limbs indicating first aid or medical attention. Two individuals had evidence of firearms injuries while six others had hard tissue damage. Despite the lack of complete body recovery, four individuals showed two or more instances of hard tissue damage. In that there were two instances in which bullets lodged in bodies it is concluded that they were not shot at close range. In no instance were limbs tied. In conclusion, all evidence suggests these individuals were battle casualties who died immediately or soon after receiving their wounds. There is no evidence they were deliberately executed. No further work at this site is recommended [end of extract from report].

Besides bone, hair, nails and quite decomposed flesh with flies and maggots, the following varieties of evidence were encountered:

- summer clothing (no turbans or sandals)
- single or double-knotted plastic sheet tied into circles (various dimensions)
- string (pocket content)
- money (Afghani notes)
- unfired cartridges (in clothing and dirt)
- one bullet in flesh
- one plastic pouch containing numerous objects
- cloth pillow amulets on cord (encircling arm or neck)

I elected to bring some of the forensic evidence back with me to Canada, not knowing how Customs at the various airports would react to bullets and grenade parts. In the event, it was not a problem. They were intrigued and cooperative.

When I told a PHR staff member of my decision to excavate partial bodies, leaving the remainder in the walls, so as to determine with statistical confidence the likely number of bodies in the whole site, this decision was critically received. On humanitarian grounds, it is not appropriate to return partial remains to families. However, in this context, which, in my naivité, I viewed as preparatory to a return visit to properly excavate the site (including the burial created by me containing the 10 sets of remains) (see below) – I thought it scientifically best to sample the site as I did (Fig. 10-15).

The Nine Wells Site

Findings at the Nine Wells Site

Dec. 16th – Today we went back to the wells. Indeed there are 9 – seven filled in; 2 show water about 25' down. Both of the latter have a stink. These could be dredged to see if bodies at bottom. I picked up evidence

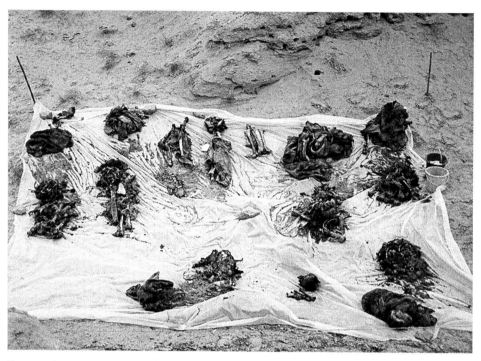

Figure 10-15. Makeshift "autopsy facility" at Dump Site: plastic sheet with remains of 10 individuals incompletely sampled.

of 3 grenades and 2 pieces of skull at the "Nine Wells" site. If Kelashnikov cartridges signal encouragement to jump down well (or direct killing) why are they lying often on surface of dirt bulldozed into well?

One person seems to have been killed for sure at this location. Could it simply be wargames area with some innocent explanation for bulldozing the wells such as poisoned water? I suppose one explanation is that the bulldozer is bulldozing up dirt and cartridges at same time. If that much firing was going on how did they avoid shooting each other? How many soldiers would be involved in forcing 100 prisoners to jump down the wells if that is indeed what happened?

The following is an extract from my report to PHR (Skinner, 1998): "This site has not been properly sampled and, yet, preliminary observations are very suggestive that improper deaths may have occurred here."

Basic well Construction. A visit to three undisturbed wells nearby, undertaken at Prof. Paik's suggestion, was very useful. Typically, the well mouth is brick-lined to depth of 2–10 metres. Depth to water at these three wells appeared to be 10–20 metres; we were told the latter depth is to be expected at the Nine Wells Site. Well mouths are approximately 1.25 m in diameter; given the depth, this is very narrow. The well mouths are incorporated into one corner of a much larger rectangular water catchment basin with brick (and internal plastic liner) or concrete walls. These are for storing the water for stock to drink (Fig. 10-16).

Forensic observations. At all nine wells, arranged basically in two irregular rows trending upslope east to west, there is one or more bulldozed tracks of disturbed earth up to 10 metres in length leading to the well mouth (see Fig. 10-5). The well mouths and basin walls are much damaged by the bulldozer. The piles of dirt pushed up at the well mouth show a light scattering of grass blades. A botanist could give a good opinion as to when the piles were created but an estimate of elapsed time of several months to less than a year would seem reasonable.

Two of the wells at the Nine Wells Site (Numbers 1 and 8) are open and yet show piled earth at the well mouth. Both have an appalling odour consistent with body decomposition. At the two open wells depth to water is about 8 metres. These too were probably plugged by bulldozed earth which has collapsed subsequently into the well. Since two wells (Numbers 4 and 6) show circular subsidence depressions to a

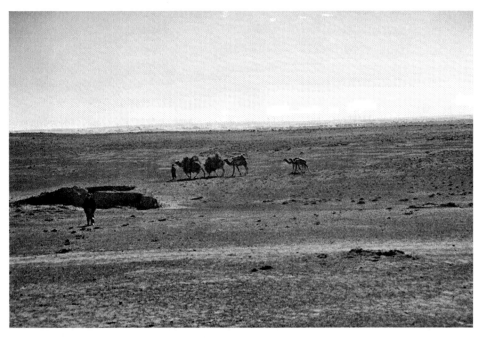

Figure 10-16. Water well and camels.

depth of 15–25 cm, clearly, the earth plug in the remaining seven wells could also collapse prior to next examination.

At all nine wells there are several to dozens of spent Kelashnikov rimless cartridges (7.62 mm × 39 mm) and one larger, rimmed "PK" cartridge (7.62 mm × 54 mm). These are on top of the basin catchment walls, within the basin or outside the walls. At well Number 8, cartridges were lying on top of the bulldozed earth piled at the well mouth. This could be explained in two ways; either the bullets had been fired after the wells had been plugged by earth (negating their forensic relevance), or the cartridges were lying on the surface around the open well mouth, but were scraped up into the bolus of earth by the bulldozer (suggesting a much larger quantity of spent cartridges was present prior to bulldozing). The latter explanation seems more credible.

There was other evidence lying on the ground surface:

1. colorful cloth fragments – especially noteworthy was a double-knotted green cloth ring found 5 metres south of Well Number 8. Three tentative diagnoses have been suggested:
    a. a wrist tie for controlling a prisoner
    b. a wrist sling (cf. Body 6 from Dump Site)
    c. armband insignia

2. grenade components were located at Well Number 7. A handle (spoon) and ring (sans pin) which were picked up from the surface; the ring was slightly buried in dirt on top of basin wall. It was of Russian manufacture. In addition, three maroon, partially threaded thick, pin-like, plastic objects about 7 cm long were observed on the surface near wells Number 3, 4 and 5. These are "transit safety plugs" from anti-personnel hand grenades. An informant at the site Dec. 10 said a grenade was thrown down the wells after the individuals were forced in.

3. two pieces of human skull bone were retrieved near Well Number 4. Both have adherent fibres. The smaller piece (?frontal) was at the margin of the earth pile plugging the well mouth while the larger (right parietal) was just outside the south wall of the basin within a metre of so of a transit plug (Fig. 10-17). The larger piece has adherent dried periosteum (soft tissue) which supports an informant's account that killings occurred within the last year. When the informant was confronted with the observation that someone had been killed above ground, rather than down the well, he responded that those reluctant to jump down the well were shot to encourage the others.

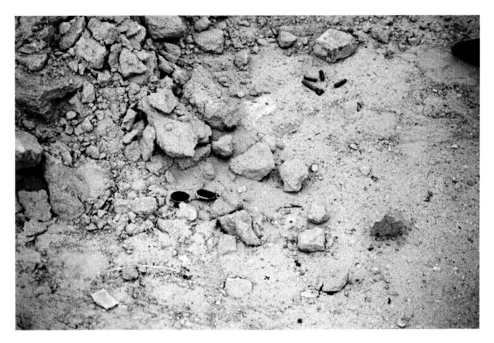

Figure 10-17. Surface evidence (scale indicated by added sunglasses): skull fragment to bottom left, transit for hand grenade and cartridge cases at top right.

Forensic Relevance of Nine Wells Site

The wells are sealed units (7 of 9) remote from any habitation. Unlike the other "mass graves" sites in northern Afghanistan they are quite undisturbed but, if one believes informant's accounts, may contain a verifiable record of behaviors which in combination qualify as a massive violation of human rights; viz:

- hundreds of victims
- Taliban soldiers
* • deaths in summer 1997
* • individuals being bound (i.e., prisoners)
* • shooting of individuals at well mouth
- individuals forced to jump down well or thrown
* • use of grenades
* • bulldozing to hide evidence
* • current evidence lends some support

---

*end of extract from report (Skinner, 1998)

UPSHOT OF ACTIVITIES, REPORTS AND RECOMMENDATIONS

Wed. Dec. 17th – I've just packed my room. I'm leaving behind shovels and implements of destruction (as Arlo Guthrie used to say) but I'm taking General Dostum's gift rug with me; so I'm still pretty laden.

Dec. 18th – Islamabad: still not sure when I can return to Canada. Spent the day checking out the physical evidence recovered from bodies and wells. Learned that fuse wire with body 5 may be trip wire from booby trap and maroon pins are from anti-personnel mines. Scary thought – whether they are above or below ground. This will make well excavation difficult if unexploded. Jean won't like this. Treated myself to mutton curry and crepes suzettes in my hotel room. At 9 PM I went out and confirmed to my relief that the 36 exp. film was OK. I wrote up a summary of my findings today and faxed them to Geneva. I've been highflying last 2 weeks. Next week back to my paper route.

Upon my return from the field, I wrote a letter to the Special Rapporteur's assistant, expressing my misgivings about the media release issued before I had undertaken any excavation. John Mills, Communications Advisor, UNHCHR, provided information on December 16, 1997 to Reuters that, in part:

A UN investigator who visited mass graves in Afghanistan discovered that hundreds of captives were thrown down wells and then killed with grenades, the United Nations rights spokesman said on Tuesday.

Local officials in the northern town of Shiberghan say mass graves in the desert contain the bodies of Taliban fighters captured last May after bitter fighting in Mazar-I-Sharif.

They were thrown into the wells either alive or those who resisted were shot and then tossed in. . . . Shots were fired into the well and hand grenades thrown in before the top of the well was bulldozed over, the spokeman added (Nebehay, 1997).

Well, this was Dostum's version; little of the above had been properly substantiated and certainly some of it was in error, in that the Dump Site was, as far as I could make out from an excavated sample, simply battle casualties. The Nine Wells Site had not been excavated to determine its contents.

In Canada, I wrote a formal report to PHR who sent a version on to the UNHCHR. I was asked to prepare a costed proposal to undertake a proper forensic investigation of the sites I had reported. I did so, estimating that it would cost about $86,000US (excluding basic supplies) for a staff of 8 persons dealing with two major sites for a period of three months.

I selected the Nine Wells Site and the Ridge Site for further analysis (as well as some single graves). Logistically, the Nine Wells site was challenging. I felt there were two optional strategies based on time and money constraints: (a) sampling several or all nine wells to obtain minimal, essential evidence for a conviction or; (b) total recovery of all evidence from one well to document the full extent of the alleged criminal behaviors. Digging the wells also presented options: dredging (easier but damaging), excavation from above (archaeologically difficult), excavation from the side (expensive but straightforward).

The Ridge Site could have been excavated in its entirety (estimated to be about 150 bodies tied in rows). Given the ease of excavation, undisturbed forensic context and excellent preservation, it was judged better to spend the majority of effort at this site. Autopsy and post-mortem examination would have been made more difficult by the mummified condition of the remains.

I was advised the budget was way too low; for example, I had neglected to provide the pathologist with an autopsy assistant. Consequently, I was told the budget was virtually doubled and forwarded to the UN where apparently the budget doubled again (for unspecified reasons) at which point the project was deemed too expensive and abandoned. Realistically, political pressures probably prevented the project from proceeding.

Two years later, when I was working in East Timor, I met a UN logistician who had managed to obtain photographs of a couple of the wells from the Nine Wells Site, dug by persons unknown, at a time unknown with unknown results. Presumably the Taliban dug the sites.

CONCLUSION

There is a distinction in cultural anthropology between "etic" and "emic"; between reach and grasp. Indeed, that is the point of this article. Usually I write articles which promote best practice in forensic archaeology (e.g., Skinner, 1987; Skinner et al., 2003). Actual practice, as shown here, may fall far short of these ideals. Good forensic archaeology (Dupras et al., 2006) as often accomplished on a domestic scale should be our goal internationally. Even if one were to overcome personal inexperience and be well-equipped, only a combination of in-depth forensic investigation, supported by sustained political will, can effectively enable forensic archaeology to be realized and to make a difference.

REFERENCES

Constable, P. (1999). A crack in the Taliban's veil. *Vancouver Sun Newspaper*. May 12:A15.

Dupras, T.L., Schultz, J.J., Wheeler, S.M., and Williams, L.J. (2006). *Forensic recovery of human remains: Archaeological approaches*. Boca Raton, CRC Press.

Dupree, L. (1997). *Afghanistan*. Karachi, Oxford University Press.

Nebehay, S. (1997). *Geneva:* Reuters.

Rubin, B.R. (1996). *The fragmentation of Afghanistan: State formation and collapse in the international system*. Lahore, Vanguard Books.

Skinner, M.F. (1987). Planning the archaeological recovery of evidence from recent mass graves. *Forensic Science International, 34*:267–287.

Skinner, M.F. Human remains from alleged mass graves in Northern Afghanistan. January 6, 1998. *Physicians for Human Rights Report submitted to United Nations High Commissioner for Human Rights*.

Skinner, M.F., Alempijevic, D., and Djuric-Srejic, M. (2003). Guidelines for international forensic bioarchaeology monitors of mass grave exhumations. *Forensic Science International, 134*:81–92.

Skinner, M.F., and Sterenberg, J. (2005). Turf wars: Authority and responsibility for the investigation of mass graves. *Forensic Science International, 151*:221–232.

Wright, R., Hanson, I., and Sterenberg, J. (2005). The archaeology of mass graves. In *Forensic archaeology: Advances in theory and practice*, Hunter, J., and Cox, M., (Eds.). London, Routledge, pp. 137–158.

Chapter 11

PREPARING THE GROUND: ARCHAEOLOGY IN A WAR ZONE

JOHN HUNTER AND BARRIE SIMPSON

BACKGROUND

Modern conflict, whether brought about by political, tribal or racial conflict, can bring with it human abuse and destruction at a scale barely comprehensible to most western societies. Death is an unfortunate but inevitable by-product of military conflict, and accepted rules apply under the articles of the Geneva Convention in terms, for example, of weaponry and treatment of civilians (e.g., United Nations 1949, Article 3). This does not excuse warfare: it is a blunt acceptance that warfare may always occur but within defined parameters of acceptability and with expected consequences. This inevitability is recognised by numerous non-governmental organisations (NGOs) with regard to post-conflict events, notably the International Commission of the Red Cross (ICRC) (2003; 2004). This is not to say that nations which ostensibly adhere to the Geneva Convention necessarily do so in the theatre of warfare, although with current media technology and embedded journalism, infringement is harder to conceal, and more embarrassing to admit.

However, conflicts which follow the Geneva Convention are effectively "official" conflicts which commence with declaration of war and conclude with cease-fire and treaty. Many other conflicts, less newsworthy because they have no recognised basis and/or occur in places remote from media interest, have neither defined starting nor end points. They play by no rules regarding weaponry, human rights abuse

266

or violation of the victims. They can, and invariably do, involve deliberate civilian rather than military slaughter on a large scale as a process of genocide or "cleansing," involving women and children as well as men of fighting age; conflicts may involve desecration of places of worship, and the razing of landscapes and burning of buildings in order to exterminate specific ethnic communities. This process only ends when one adversary or community has been effectively erased by the other or when third party intervention (e.g., the United Nations) occurs, otherwise the conflict and the death continue to simmer.

In either case, the magnitude of conflict is measured by victim numbers, in thousands or in tens of thousands, but the difference between condoned warfare and civil conflict and genocide is manifest most in the treatment of individuals and in the disposal of the dead. The Geneva Convention accords dignity to the victims through appropriate burial and repatriation (United Nations, 1977); (see Chapter 2 of this volume on international law). Outside this Convention, anything goes according to convenience and profit: victims can be tipped into machine-dug mass graves having been executed at the grave edge or elsewhere; they can be dropped into wells or mine shafts, or wedged into caves. The process is one of concealment in order to prevent detection rather than disposal for reverential purposes; the aim is to remove from sight rather than to commemorate. Avoidance of identification may entail these human remains to be burnt, disarticulated by explosives, or booby-trapped to inhibit recovery. Some graves are known to have been re-excavated by the perpetrators and the victims reburied in secondary graves through fear of detection. And there is the additional factor of those graves which have been created not by perpetrators, but by families and relatives who gathered the dead together for more venerated disposal. In their own way, these may also constitute "mass graves" but here the intention is to respect the individuals rather than simply dispose of evidence, and to commemorate their interment rather than conceal their whereabouts. There is much in common here with burial of many of the Indonesian *Tsunami* victims of 2004 where individuals were buried for environmental, hygienic and storage reasons by official agencies or by communities.

The participation of archaeologists and anthropologists in the investigation of any of these types of graves was, even in the 1980s, not always considered necessary in a process that was perceived as one of straightforward exhumation. Since then, the importance of recovering forensic evidence and ensuring proper identification has required a more skilled approach than the simple use of machine backhoes and numbered body bags (e.g., Connor and Scott, 2001). This development placed anthropologists and archaeologists in a largely unfamiliar context, not least with regard to the nature of their "raw material," evidential requirements, scale of operation, security, and a host of other factors relevant to working in a hostile environment. It is important to stress the relative newness of this situation as it became applied in Iraq: experience was still being built-up; limitations exposed (Komar, 2003); techniques and processes adapted (Skinner et al., 2003; Wright et al., 2005); new areas of expertise recognised (e.g., Haglund, 2002) and the nature of evidence, notably the recognition of human rights abuse, was becoming better appreciated (Steadman and Haglund, 2005).

A stage has been reached by which standard operating procedures (SOPs) and protocols could be defined, although these have to be seen as "snapshots" in the evolution of learning and understanding, rather than as absolutes. SOPs and protocols are documents for fair weather; they are idealised statements of how things should be done and why they should be done, but all tend to be less adaptable than the work allows. They need to be flexible not only to natural environment and physical circumstance, as in any archaeological scenario, but also to political situation, the presence of grieving relatives and, most significantly, to the imposition of an organisational authority for which archaeological and anthropological intervention may sometimes be accepted for cosmetic purposes only.

There is the corollary to this too: namely that failure of investigations to adhere to the idealised guidance of defined SOPs and complex protocols may jeopardise any subsequent legal proceedings. But this, of course, depends on the nature of contemporary social values, the justice system involved, and the political environment in which the scenario is brought to justice. We are accustomed to believe that western (i.e., UK and US) standards are the appropriate standards to apply worldwide, but that fails to take into account local values, traditional justice systems, and ethnic and religious beliefs within societies for whom UK and US attitudes of justice may be neither appropriate nor relevant (Hunter and Cox, 2005:207).

Much debate has existed for several years on "minimum standards," SOPs and protocols. There is no internationally recognised standard, beyond that of the basic guidelines issued by the United Nations (1991) known as the "The Minnesota Protocol," and although many international forensic organisations each have their own versions, there are more similarities than differences. The differences, apart from the change in logo or copyright, are mainly in the fine detail, and all seek adequately to satisfy the basic requirements of a Court, along the lines required by the United Nations for their Tribunals in Rwanda and in the former Yugoslavia.

Post-conflict and insurgency-active areas present difficult and dangerous theatres of operations with problems of physical, political and logistical natures. In these situations, field operatives require clear and simple guidelines to achieve the desired result, enabling them to work both effectively and efficiently within local constraints to the satisfaction of their contracting organisation. There is an operational need to separate what is *essential* from what is *desirable* and to create a working set of minimum standards, clearly and simply stating what is necessary at a site to achieve the desired result. The basic requirements outlined by the United Nations in "The Minnesota Protocol" are already proven to be internationally acceptable to a court. Anything beyond could be viewed as an enhancement. By its very nature, forensic work requires flexibility and adaptability from site-to-site, (e.g., Hoshower, 1998); rigid adherence to sets of conditions and guidelines which constrain this flexibility may also constrain the results.

Archaeologists and anthropologists may sometimes find themselves in very deep water: they may not be in control of the working environment in which they operate; their roles may not be fully recognised by other evidential agencies (see Skinner and Sterenberg, 2005); the standards to which they work may necessarily fall short of their own professional expectations, and the judicial system may be wholly alien to their own experience. Archaeologists and anthropologists working in a war zone must recognise not only the potential value of their contribution, but also the severe limitations that may apply.

There are ethical issues here, too. Is it better to provide support in a limited way, even if there is little control over the output of events and data, on the basis that it is better to do something rather than nothing? Or is it better to reject a role in a scenario because the methodology is likely to be sub-standard (from a western viewpoint) or the outcome unacceptable? And does it make a difference if the judicial authority in question legitimises capital punishment, as in Iraq? These questions are real and have been faced by archaeologists and anthropologists working in theatre. It would be naive to believe that archaeology in a war zone can be undertaken as a straightforward scientific programme of investigation with the same political and judicial security as that enjoyed, for example, in the UK.

This is not new. Mass graves have been dug before, and the learning experience continues (see Stover and Ryan, 2001). The processes are not novel and both theoretical approaches and practical shortcomings have begun to appear in literature, but only in the reporting of individual mass graves, in particular techniques employed, or in general advice given (e.g., Haglund et al., 2001). This is not to be critical, but to reflect the learning curve of excavating mass graves. Papers tend to be about technical specifics: there is little yet in the way of overview; the effects of excavation strategy on judicial outcomes, or on placing mass graves in the wider historical context of genocide.

We are watching the development of a discipline in its formative, sometimes clumsy, growth in which its eager practitioners are sometimes uncertain of their role, lack confidence in their abilities, and have few mentors for reassurance. Because the discipline is so young it lacks the age and experience profile of most other disciplines: the practitioners are generally young (20–35) and have largely developed the discipline themselves, and there is little in the way of either career structure or elders to provide benchmark and guidance. These practitioners work according to ability, commonsense and conscience.

Much of this work is arguably processual, but every archaeologist needs to respond to questions asked – the dynamic that charges academic enquiry – rather than the clinical deconstruction of a mass burial. The two are not the same. It is the questioning of these remains that fuels the investigative process, and one of the primary aspects of any war zone archaeology is to establish which graves are being targeted, why they are being targeted, and what questions are being asked. This is no different from a research design which assesses the sites available in order to determine those which are best suited to respond to the questions posed. Selection might favour graves which best reflect human rights abuse, graves for which named military figures or individuals can be associated for conviction purposes, graves known to contain particular groups of victims from a particular community or with a particular ethnic or religious affiliation, or graves constructed at a specific time according to aerial imagery. The existence of eye-witness accounts might give some graves additional forensic weight.

The nature of some of these questions can sometimes be ostensibly straightforward. When were these victims killed? How were they killed? Were they killed at the grave side? Are the victims soldiers or are they civilians? Did human rights abuse take place? The time and attention paid to the investigation of a single murder victim in (for example) the UK will not be multiplied by the number of victims excavated from a mass grave. The questions are more likely to be generic than individualised, although aspects of individualisation may occur when (or if) identification processes and DNA analysis takes place. Some practitioners find this concentration of process distasteful, but it is a matter of practicality and best use of resources rather than deliberate inhumanity.

Legal proceedings may simply need to know that a group of persons (men, women and children) from a particular location (A) have disappeared and have been discovered in a mass grave in another location (B). This simple level of information, even as a sample, may be deemed sufficient to instigate proceedings against a particular military individual held to be responsible. This may be the focus of the questioning, but it should not inhibit the archaeologists and anthropologists from making a full analysis and record of all evidence available. Archaeology is destructive and there are strong ethical issues involved in investigations of this type; there is no guarantee that the excavated evidence may not need to be reviewed in the future in order to respond to different forensic questions.

PRACTICALITIES

Archaeologists and anthropologists operating within a war zone need to establish before departure under whose authority they will be acting. In an immediate post-conflict environment there will be an official, if temporary, "Provisional Government," possibly under the flag of the United Nations, as in the former Yugoslavia, or a military-political coalition, as was the situation in 2003–2004 within Iraq. There will also be a number of NGOs, all acting for the benefit of the surviving community as their main objective, but often with differing aims. Their methodologies or emphases may also differ, and even sometimes from that of the provisional government.

Forensics, by definition, act in support of a legal authority. Without direct and written lawful authority the activities are *per se* non-forensic and potentially illegal in a subsequent court of law. Similarly, humanitarian missions likewise require "lawful authority." Engagement by a governing authority, even one of a temporary nature, also by definition will legitimise any archaeological intervention; engagement by an NGO (and this includes most international forensic organisations that operate within this sphere) will only legitimise activities if the NGO in question is formally recognised or approved by the governing authority.

Formal authority has a direct impact on the level of personal security. This is a high priority in the hostile environment of a post-conflict theatre, particularly if armed insurgency remains an active threat. Personal safety, movements and forensic work depend totally on the level of security provided (also see Chapter 3 of this volume). Operations contracted by a governing authority will normally include military protection, or the provision of a good standard of armed private security. Operations contracted by an NGO may differ, given the variable standards of private security companies: some employ highly professional former Special Forces personnel with appropriate training and equipment; others use the services of "local security" of undefined standard, ability and experience.

During the initial forensic mission undertaken in Iraq between 2003–2004 under the authority of the Coalition Provisional Authority (CPA), a military liaison officer was permanently attached to the small CPA Forensic Team to facilitate military security requirements. In many ways this highlights the need to act under "lawful authority." It guaranteed that the team's security would be either from one of the Coalition Military Units or private security firms of a highly professional competency, with all the necessary equipment, communications and (importantly) experienced and highly trained staff provided by one of the Coalition Provisional Governments. In Iraq, this was provided to UK staff by a private security firm contracted by the UK Foreign and Commonwealth Office.

These are security issues specific to the investigation in question. There are other security factors of broader nature, notably threats posed by "stray" explosives and mines. Personnel working in theatre are supported with (obligatory) advice and guidance on unexploded ordnance (UXO), types of munitions and weaponry, and the function of EOD (Explosive Ordnance Disposal) teams. Mine awareness courses are well-established on forensic missions; they usually commence on arrival at the destination airport even in the early hours of the morning. In

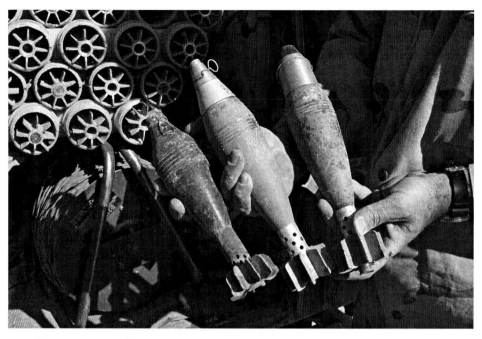

Figure 11-1. A selection of live ammunition found by EOD personnel in Iraq.

Iraq, there was the continual discovery of unexploded ordnance of all types, from actual weapons varying from small arms to rocket-propelled grenade launchers and unexploded mines, to shells and munitions of all calibres (Fig. 11-1). Many of these were often first discovered by the forensic team during their daily tasks.

Security is essential but restrictive. While the forensic archaeologist retains responsibility for site selection and visits, decisions regarding where and when travel takes place are vested with the security team, either military or private. Personnel are at their most vulnerable during movement within a hostile environment. This has been highlighted in Iraq and Afghanistan with the use of improvised explosive devices (IEDs), ambushes on convoys, and kidnapping incidents. Ostensibly simple logistics involved in moving a forensic team are often difficult to undertake and need to be recognised. Moving two forensic archaeologists from a secure military base to a suspect site in Iraq involved an ongoing in-depth intelligence and threat level assessment on both the suspected area and the routes to and from the site; it also required the provision of an armed security escort of an officer and 12 soldiers with six armoured vehicles (Fig. 11-2) (all of which provided the security

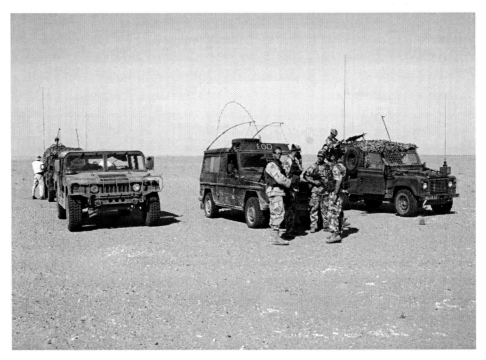

Figure 11-2. Part of the security convoy required by any forensic mission in Iraq.

perimeter while work was taking place on the site), an EOD team (two more soldiers and vehicle), and a field ambulance (two military paramedics and vehicle). Some sites are only safely accessed by helicopter entailing similarly difficult travel logistics. The complexities of any travel method demonstrate the necessity of maintaining a military liaison presence within the forensic team itself. When on the site there must also be an acceptance that the time available for the archaeologist to undertake an assessment is dependent on the knowledge of the security commander, not of the archaeologist.

There may be real threat to life and limb in some environments, and contingency needs to be made in case something goes wrong on a mission. This is not a case of lost luggage or travel delay (both of which are almost inevitable) but of worst possible scenarios. Missions to an immediate post-conflict or insurgency-active environment require carefully defined levels of insurance, for both life and injury, with linked medical care and medical evacuation provision as necessary. Activities in hostile environments may almost certainly negate existing domestic life cover policies, and with them associated benefits for mortgages and dependants. Very few insurance companies offer "off the peg" cover for working in a conflict zone; cover will be bespoke and with high premiums which can rise exponentially with levels of hostile activities within the theatre of operation. In 2004, an insurance policy for working in such an environment (Iraq) for cover for loss of life, injury and medical evacuation was £7,000 GBP for a three-month period.

The threat assessment is a constant; it can result in all the planning to visit a site being cancelled at short notice, and hence, one practical solution is always to have alternative sites to visit; remembering that even those alternatives may not be possible. Cancellation can even occur during the actual journey to the site or while on the site itself prompting an immediate withdrawal. Security is an essential factor not only for the archaeologists and anthropologists concerned, but also for the accompanying military personnel. Security apart, their very presence with the archaeologists removes them from other tasks. Moreover, they may be taking on additional duties in order to support the forensic team.

Experience suggests that forensic missions can be broken down into five main phases of interrelated activity: the public awareness phase; the site assessment phase; the excavation phase; the postmortem phase, and the repatriation phase. All need to be taken into account, planned and properly resourced in advance. There is a strong logistical and ethical argument to suggest that unless the practicalities of all five can be met securely, then the mission should not take place at all.

This was the approach adopted in Iraq by the initial CPA Forensic Team during 2003–2004. There are difficulties within this approach in that there are pressures on the initial forensic team, despite its size (which in Iraq was just four personnel), to "dig." The team may, therefore, spend a great deal of time and effort in negotiating with local communities and explaining to the Governing Authority precisely what is involved in a full scale excavation and examination process. Both expect instant results, often above and beyond what can be practically or forensically achieved.

Underpinning these activities were the logistics which involved identifying and obtaining the proper equipment required for full-scale excavations and postmortem processes, the identification of mortuary facilities, both temporary and permanent, and obtaining sufficient staffing levels, with all the attendant issues of availability and accommodation. These are complex logistics requiring careful preparation; this is an arena for professionalism, not for "do-gooding." The following sections outline some of the principal themes and issues. Greater detail can be found elsewhere (e.g., Wright et al., 2005) and in the various SOPs and protocols according to mission (e.g., CPA, 2003; ICTY, 2001).

PUBLIC AWARENESS

Some execution and burial sites may already be known to surviving local populations. Initial and understandable reactions are for survivors and relatives to take it upon themselves to recover the victims – an action which has perhaps long been denied to them. In post-conflict Iraq there were many scenes, some televised worldwide, of local communities excavating mass grave sites. Opinions differ as to the ethics of this. On one hand, forensic scientists argue that this community-led process destroys evidence of criminal acts and jeopardises conclusive personal identification; on the other hand, there is an equally valid argument to question the right of the international community to deny the survivors their right to recover their loved ones. Scientific reasoning holds small sway in such an emotive situation.

Not all such occurrences may result from the disorganised reaction of an emotive local community. Many local exhumations have been led by community leaders such as doctors and lawyers who maintained basic records of recoveries and repatriations to families without the "advantages" of advice from forensic scientists. This was clearly evidenced within parts of Iraq, for example, at the initial "community exhumation" of a known mass grave site at Hillah. In this case, the media coverage led to a perception by the forensic community in the West of complete disorganisation, whereas in reality much was being done to record and identify by local medical practitioners. To impose an alternative strategy without explanation is guaranteed to lose the sympathy of the very people whose support is essential, especially if a time delay needs to be built into the excavation programme.

A programme of public awareness is an essential element of forensic process in this environment (Fig. 11-3). It establishes an honest awareness of the benefits of in-depth investigation and the value of waiting for a full forensic team to undertake the exhumations on the community's behalf. The problem with public awareness programmes is satisfying the needs of these surviving communities by producing tangible results within a time delay that is acceptable to the local community.

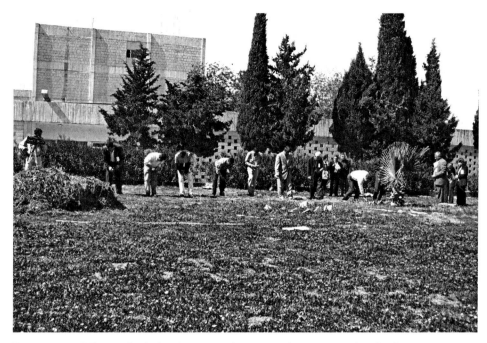

Figure 11-3. What to look for. Line search training being given by the forensic team to local personnel in Iraq.

Investigating teams are in the hands of the governing authority or NGO, or even the international political community on whom the archaeologist relies for the provision of the finance, staff and logistics. There is rarely a direct relationship between the archaeologists and anthropologists and the community in question, if only through language difficulties. Instead the relationship is indirect; there is inevitably an intermediary, or some organisational or administrative third party involved, or even military, which can inadvertently generate a strained operational environment.

The creation of local awareness also chimes well with the provision of capacity building. Relationships may benefit from the involvement of members of local communities in awareness programmes, for example, on excavation processes, postmortem examination, crime scene methods and evidence handling. This might be particularly relevant to local medical personnel and lawyers. In Iraq, several of these awareness sessions, held by the forensic team over two or three days, were undertaken in various locations around the country, although in no way did they replace the desire for action and involvement by the surviving communities. But they did provide an element of local participation, and they did much to diminish the perception of "colonialism" that internationalism tends to foster. In the Balkans, local archaeologists have been trained in the skills of excavating mass graves in the anticipation that at some point in the future these sites can be managed and excavated to the required standards by home-grown nationals.

SITE ASSESSMENT

One of the first major practical tasks to be undertaken by archaeologists and anthropologists in a forensic response team is the creation of a centralised database of reported or suspected mass grave sites. Experience in both the Balkans and in Iraq has demonstrated the importance of this: sites were known to the military, local community groups as well as to NGOs, and in Iraq the total list of sites was numbered in hundreds, between them containing thousands of victims. The creation of a centralised database identified much duplication, many suspected sites being listed several times under different names in the same location. There may also be associated lists of missing persons. Often in the immediate post-conflict period persons are reported as "missing" to a variety of agencies or NGOs and this, like the identification of suspect sites, can lead to duplication and distortion of figures. Lists of "the missing" need to be centralised if they are to be reliable. Some NGOs specialise in the provision of this type of information, notably the ICRC.

In Iraq, this centralised site database was identified by the forensic response team as an urgent forensic priority. It had full support of the CPA and the invaluable assistance of a computer database which the International Commission on Missing Persons (ICMP) allowed the forensic team to use. As a result, an accurate identification of suspected mass grave sites could take place.

The team was also supported in its desire to establish a centralised database for "the missing." This was part of a longer term objective for identification and repatriation (below) and beyond the normal remit of archaeologists and anthropologists but, during the immediate post-conflict period when there were no investigators in place, the team found itself wearing many hats. Again, the CPA was supportive of the Missing Persons initiative and this was pursued within the fledgling Iraqi Ministry of Human Rights.

Subject to the restrictions imposed by security and logistics, all suspected sites required first-hand inspection and assessment by experienced archaeologists in order to confirm status. This process could often be difficult to arrange for logistical and security reasons, but was an important step in creating an accurate assessment of mass grave integrity and location. An initial assessment involved minimal investigative and recording activity, but needed much in the way of common sense and experience in recognising disturbed ground and landscape change.

The choice of which grave to address, and why, can only result effectively from the undertaking of audit. The mission needed to verify the number of graves available for investigation, and identify those which best answered the questions being posed within the constraints of access and security, and according to the many variables which might apply. Not least of these is that of size. Curiously, there is no single accepted definition of a mass grave; Skinner (1987) talks of more than half a dozen bodies while the UN (1991) talks of three or more. A working definition might consider, for example:

- Single grave   1 body
- Multiple grave   2–5 bodies
- Mass grave   6 or more bodies

The above was created and applied by the CPA Forensic Team for Iraq. This simple and practical working definition provoked more discussion among practitioners outside theatre than the success of the assessment process being initiated. As argued above, there is need to create a working set of minimum standards and definitions, clearly and simply stating what is necessary at a site to achieve the desired result, not an academic debate.

Each site needs to be considered on its merits in a standardised process and in Iraq the initial team created a Standardised Assessment Guide in a simple booklet format with the basic requirements: a ten figure grid reference; a correct name (together with all known alternative local names); a health and safety site review including EOD assessment; overhead imagery (satellite and aerial); maps (local and international); site geophysical survey (if available); details of any invasive survey undertaken; site survey plans; site sketch plans; digital photographs and photographic log sheet; anthropological assessment of any surface remains (occasionally of remains in any trial trench); exhibit lists of any artefacts recovered; and details of any potential witnesses encountered.

At this early stage the forensic team might coincidentally generate further intelligence such as witness information, or artefacts in the form of bullet cases or human material lying adjacent to suspected sites. These needed to be logged accordingly in order to demonstrate proper continuity. Even by this stage the bureaucratic trail has already started; the paperwork, pro-formas and logging mechanisms were prepared in advance and linked into the centralised database. In essence, even the primary audit of potential sites brings with it commitment.

It thus became possible to deploy basic archaeological techniques to site identification and to produce an accurate evaluation quite separate from any reliance on rumour and second-hand information. Assessments such as these are an essential element of primary process and can be undertaken successfully by a small team with minimal equipment starting with "desktop" analysis, typically using aerial or satellite imagery supported by Geographical Information Systems (GIS). The obtaining of accurate information also has the benefit of smoothing the subsequent forensic process into the excavation and postmortem stages. The deployment, for example, of geophysical survey and 3-D imaging of data may generate a broad picture of size, depth and capacity of grave with resource implications for the numbers of excavation and autopsy staff required, the time needed to excavate, and the facilities required (Hunter et al., 2005). Assessment ensures that scarce resources of time and money can be directed effectively and efficiently to known sites where the best or primary evidence is most likely to be obtained.

Iraq had not only a high number of reported mass grave sites and missing persons, but was also of a sheer geographical size that made moving teams and equipment difficult – factors compounded by a harsh physical environment and security dangers. In liaison with the CPA, it was decided during the assessment phase to prioritise the identification of a number of specific mass graves which would provide evidence of the seven major known periods of Human Rights atrocity. These were defined as being: the 1980 Persecution of the Faylee Kurds; the 1983 Kurdish Massacres against the Barzanis/KDP (Kurdistan Democratic Party); the 1988 Anfal Campaign; the 1988 chemical attack on Halabja; the 1991 Shi'a Uprising; the 1991 Kurdish Autonomy; and the 1999 Uprising in Najaf. The purpose of this was to establish a priority list of undisturbed sites which would reflect examples of each of the major periods of atrocity, in order to maximise the resources that would subsequently be deployed for full forensic excavations.

One of the graves identified (unnamed here for security reasons) provides a useful example of some of the issues that arose. It was a desert site containing multiple mass graves where the initial assessment was restricted to a single period of thirty minutes for security reasons. Nevertheless, this was sufficient time to gather the necessary essential data using the team's Standardised Assessment Guide that would allow enquiries to continue. Subsequently, desktop research took place using military intelligence reports, mapping and aerial imagery; this included dated satellite spectral images which could identify when disturbances had occurred in the geological matrix of the desert floor.

This primary visit had been undertaken under security provided by the UK military but, due to changes in areas of responsibility, the second visit required negotiations with another Coalition Military member, the Netherlands. In addition, the team had to negotiate air transport by Hercules from Baghdad to another military airfield and then a Chinook helicopter from that airfield to the nearest military base to the site. Once more, the security arrangements required to move the two forensic archaeologists from the secure military base to the site entailed continuous intelligence and threat assessments on both the suspected area and the routes to and from the site, and the provision of six armoured vehicles, EOD team and field ambulance as previously supplied.

On this second occasion a more detailed assessment was possible. The whole site was planned, recorded and photographed. A trial trench excavated across one of the suspected graves exposed the depth to the top of the body mass and provided sufficient evidence to support the site as being representative of one of the known periods of atrocity (Fig. 11-4). The evidence was fully documented and the location of the trial trench precisely recorded by Global Positioning System (GPS) before the trench was back-filled. It was noted on this second visit that a few dry shrubs were growing on the graves and that two graves appeared to be linked by a shallow and narrow gully which was possible due to the result of water action. Contrary to popular belief it does rain, although infrequently, in a desert environment, specifically in the winter period. Hunter et al. (1996:87) have discussed the extremes of burial type and the effects which the burial of human remains may have on associated vegetational growth – factors which were tested further by helicopter in this desert environment to determine whether the distribution of these shrubs might be diagnostic of graves during the winter "rainy period." From the air each of the individual graves on this multiple

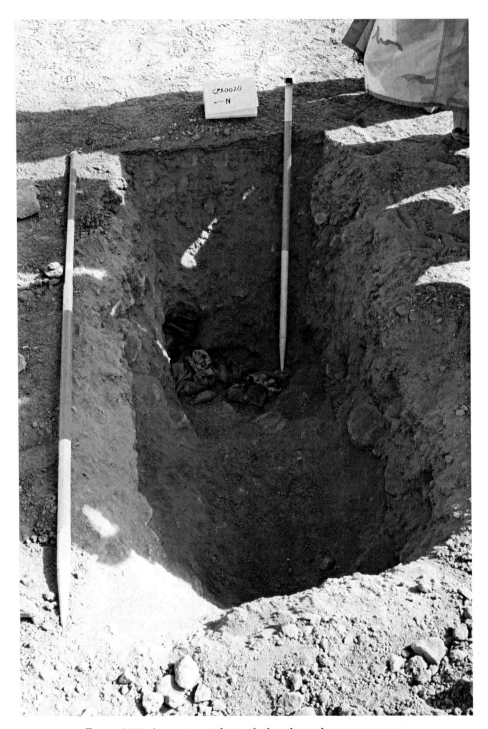

Figure 11-4. A narrow trial trench dug through a suspect area.

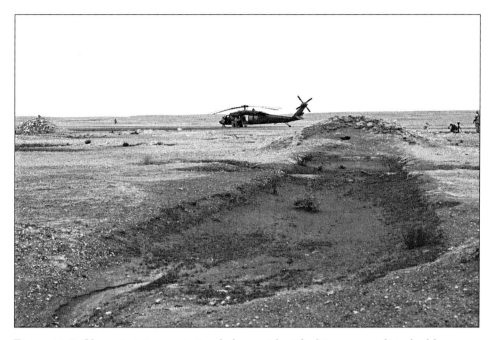

Figure 11-5. Characteristic vegetational change identified in an area disturbed by grave construction.

mass grave site were disclosed as green oblong shapes against the surrounding desert environment (Fig. 11-5). The phenomenon allowed an optimum timeframe to be identified for aerial survey, notably during the winter months, December–February, in such desert locations as exist in Iraq.

This assessment process, involving the obtaining of minimal and essential information, was successfully repeated at a number of other sites across Iraq. It was initially undertaken by the response team and subsequently on other sites using consistent documentation by other small national teams from Denmark and Finland.

EXCAVATION

Once a priority list of appropriate sites has been drawn up, there is often likely to be strong pressure exerted on the archaeologists to start the excavation process. These demands will almost certainly be made by officials who have little or no idea of what archaeology is about, how evidence is gathered and recorded, or how long it takes. Much time will be spent explaining the exact nature of the work involved and the logistics required. There is a process of "mission" involved here; it may be continually repeated as new personnel or professionals with different evidential requirements move in. All will need to be made aware that excavation is destructive and therefore that time and meticulous examination are essential requisites to ensure that maximum evidence is recovered. Equally, the archaeologists and anthropologists need to be aware of the work of others working on the same scene, and of the security implications of the work required. To undertake any forensic process in circumstances that could be interrupted by hostile action, lead to its abandonment as incomplete, or even lead to the unnecessary threat to the life and limb of the investigator, is creating a self-defeating process for both the surviving victims seeking closure and for the legal process seeking justice.

Not only are activities in respect of excavation limited by hostilities, they also depend heavily on adequate preparation. In an immediate post-conflict period neither the necessary staff, nor the equipment required for the excavation phase of a mass grave of, for example 300 victims, nor the logistics for the creation and staffing of a mortuary for the postmortem examination phase will immediately be in place. Outline facilities require an electricity supply for equipment and body storage facilities, water for washing remains (and drinking), fuel for transport, not to mention security, food, shelter and accommodation for the participants. In remote, rural or desert situations these ostensibly basic facilities may require complex logistics. Working in a hostile environment may also entail living in a country with a ruined infrastructure and limited supply lines. There will also be other pressing demands for facilities and financial resources from other components of any restructuring programme. To place this in perspective, even with a full team, full logistical support and security, the current US-led team still operating in Iraq has only excavated two sites, and not fully completed those, at the time of writing.

On a practical level, excavation presents many options of approach and solution according to questions asked. Practical methodology may be biased towards "plinth" or more standard "open trench" excavation according to the nature of soils, water table and climate (e.g., Wright et al., 2005). Other options may necessitate sampling or "slicing" – a process in which part of a mass grave is excavated and a sample of the victims recovered. This might be used to demonstrate how "x" number of victims died, and to provide a breakdown percentage of the sex, age, stature and ethnicity of those sampled, from which an inference is drawn in respect of the remainder of the victims. In theory this allows evidence to be obtained rapidly in a hostile environment and used to support a tribunal, but it also presents wider ethical considerations. Furthermore, analysis of fully excavated mass graves suggests that sampling might easily provide misleading data (see Wright et al., 2005, Figure 5.2).

MORTUARY INFRASCTRUCTURE

Once the recovery of human remains or artefacts commences, the key issue is that of maintaining the continuity of evidence, the so-called "chain of custody." The movement of all human remains and associated artefacts from grave to mortuary should accord to an existing process of preplanning and record, not to an *ad hoc* manoeuvre according to availability of personnel and facility at the time. Furthermore, the information needed for permanent archive requires that all processes should adhere to a predefined system of documentation amenable to storage and re-evaluation. This needs to be well-thought-out in advance, not in retrospect.

In an immediate post-conflict zone or where hostile insurgency is active, little full-scale forensic excavation will be occurring as was the situation in Iraq in 2003–2004 and is still the situation there in 2007. This is the opportune time to put the machinery of mortuary facilities in place. In the same way that the creation of a centralised database and a scientific site assessment is essential for collating accurate information on suspected sites ahead of excavation, so the preparatory aspect for the mortuary and later repatriation processes is likewise essential; this will ensure that the results of that excavation are processed to standards acceptable to the courts.

For most operations in a hostile environment appropriate facilities will simply not be available, and in many instances temporary facilities will have to be created. The security situation itself may be the determining factor as to permanent or temporary mortuaries, but both will require the same level of planning and logistics to ensure appropriate security, transport, body storage, and levels of equipment and staffing to cope with the throughput. The facility will need secure and refrigerated storage for remains entering the process, and similar storage arrangement after autopsy, with an intervening area where radiography, pathology, DNA sampling and anthropology (including odontology) can take place (refer to Chapters 5 and 6 in this volume for further information).

Running parallel with these basic work requirements will be further requirements for: "clean" areas for staff to change; showers, rest, report writing; equipment storage and secure storage for any records or evidence. Many autopsies have been successfully, but not ideally, achieved in converted buildings, sheds and tents using makeshift storage facilities and trestle tables. In Kosovo, a very successful mortuary was established within a disused factory in 2000 and again in 2002; it subsequently became a permanent mortuary facility for forensic work.

Tents are usually necessary in remote or rural locations. Some may simply serve to keep the weather and prying eyes away, but others can be more sophisticated. The Swedish Government successfully deployed several with air conditioning and/or heating in extremes of temperatures in places such as the cold of an Afghan winter or heat of Iraq, where they were deployed after the bombing of the UN Headquarters in Baghdad in 2003. In Thailand, following the *Tsunami* of 2004, the Norwegian Government provided a portable prefabricated self-build mortuary system, which consisted of interconnecting single storied buildings, each the size of a large portacabin, in which several "post-mortem lines" could be operated (see Figures 11-6 and 11-7).

The initial team in Iraq was faced with this basic question of finding appropriate mortuary facilities. Existing mortuaries in the centres of population were not suitable for the logistical demands which the excavation of a mass grave would bring, and indeed were already extremely busy with dealing with the daily results of the insurgency and continued civil bombings. A new series of mortuaries set up on a regional basis was considered, but the problem here was not one of finding suitable buildings, but of the simple logistical problems of maintaining a communications infrastructure and the uninterrupted provision of power. This was a problem compounded by difficulties in ensuring a constant supply of consumables and equipment. Iraq has a single sea port, limited air heads which were essentially military bases, and a road infrastructure under constant threat of attack. The proposed solution was to adopt the temporary mortuary concept within a tented

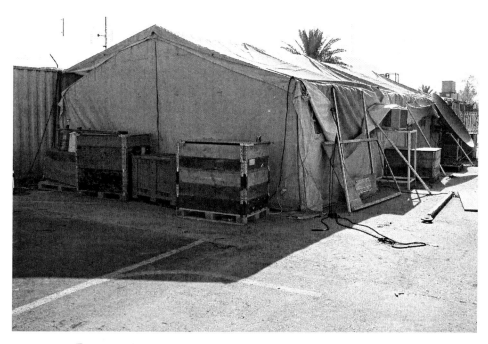

Figure 11-6. A temporary mortuary tenting arrangement in Iraq.

system working alongside, and parallel to, the excavation. The Swedish system (above) was the most viable option and allowed the full logistics and security for both the recovery and identification phases to be contained within a single site.

An efficient autopsy system may also help support a local awareness programme, and go some way to show the value of the full forensic system for obtaining evidence and forensic identification. Where a local community has already "excavated" a mass grave, then the identification is likely to have been of a presumptive nature on the basis of identity cards with (or tenuously associated with) a body, or by clothing which may not have been seen by relatives for many years since the victim's disappearance. DNA may be greeted with suspicion for a variety of reasons with a cultural or religious basis, or through simple distrust and lack of understanding. Identification by DNA is a useful preliminary liaison topic and can involve both the governing authority and local community leaders. There is no point in taking DNA samples from victims unless there is a parallel (or proposed) community outreach

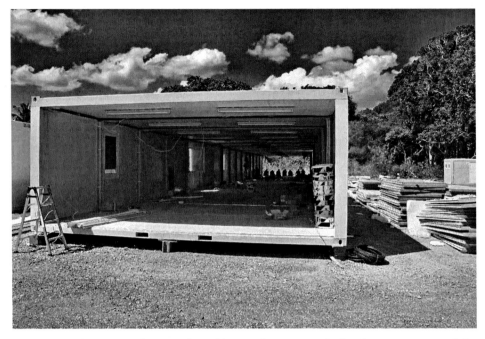

Figure 11-7. A more sophisticated prefabricated mortuary facility being constructed for the Tsunami.

programme of sampling families for the potential matching of profiles. The (re)burial of victims of the Srebrenica massacre in the Balkans is the direct result of a DNA matching programme undertaken by the ICMP which has enabled the remains to be named and returned to their families.

REPATRIATION

The interest of local communities is not necessarily in the forensic acquisition of primary data for criminal conviction, but for the return of lost relatives. Both aspects will feature as the archaeologist's and anthropologist's aims at the onset of the investigations. Repatriation may be for other than emotive reasons: without proof of death in some cultures a woman cannot marry again, and without a family she and other widows may have to live outside the normal society. Often a pension or death payment may be dependent on proof of a death. The definition of what establishes identity is a national, not a local, decision irrespective of the differences between positive and presumptive identification methodologies.

Positive identification can be achieved via DNA, fingerprints, odontology, dentures/prosthetics, medical records including x-rays, and individualising skeletal markers. By contrast, presumptive identification is usually based on personal identification cards or documents, personal effects, and clothing. The weight of scientific theory is heavily in favour of positive identification factors, but assumes integrity of data which can only be guaranteed by proper archaeological recovery. It can also rely heavily on existing dental and medical records which in many parts of the world are non-existent. Equally, clothing can sometimes be diagnostic, being worn, patched and "individualised" through poverty, and easily recognisable by a wife or mother. Presumptive identification, however, discounts the likelihood that clothes may have been changed or contents of pockets switched.

This final phase of the investigation, in the processing of post-excavation data for any prosecution, and in the identification and repatriation of the "missing" is where forensic and humanitarian issues may come into conflict, and where the success in creating an environment of public understanding will be seen most acutely. Individual bodies or body parts cannot be returned to either families or local community representative without appropriate authority, or without completion of the investigative and identification process. Sometimes this can take months.

Where an agreement is reached with the governing authority regarding the chosen method of identification, arrangements can be put in train for the return of the remains. Where only DNA identification is accepted, there will be a necessity to establish large refrigerated storage facilities for remains until a matching DNA profile is established. Only then can the remains be returned to the family for burial. In the event of the governing authority accepting presumptive identification, repatriation can be made more immediately. However, in the case of unidentified victims, body parts or commingled elements, but where the locale can be pinpointed from the identification of others in the same grave, the remains may be justifiably returned to the community in question for communal burial. There is a strong argument here for this to take place in a carefully surveyed and recorded burial area with a unique referencing numbering system. There may be occasions when the original DNA samples from these remains may be matched in the future; they may need to be identified and exhumed for any subsequent reburial.

ENDNOTE

Archaeology in a hostile environment such as post-conflict Iraq brings its own idiosyncratic problems, not least of which are the safety and security of the investigating personnel, an increased emphasis on preparation and planning, and an understanding of social and political climates at both national and local levels. The success of the mission will probably depend on the ability to make the right choices of graves for investigation, to answer the questions posed, and to gain the respect of the local community. There are no short cuts; there is no "by-the-book" method of excavating mass graves, and there is no quick way of building relationships with a grieving community. What may be a project with defined beginning and endpoints for the archaeologist and anthropologist has an immeasurably more significant effect on members of the local community. For them the excavation will be just one stage in a sequence of life-changing events. For the investigation team, there will be not only the recognition of this, but also of its awkward conciliation with the objectives of scientific enquiry – a position rarely encountered in "normal" criminal investigation.

When the excavation is over, the bodies repatriated or stored, and/or the forensic evidence drawn together for prosecution report, there will be need for proper archiving. Perhaps the discipline of excavating mass graves is too young to recognise the significance of this, and of the importance of retaining data and making it accessible. Graves and their excavation records tend to be considered in isolation for criminal purposes, and each individual victim tends to be treated separately for identification and repatriation. However, there is a wider picture that is seen neither in the evidence selected for courts nor in individual victim repatriation. The overview of different graves and different individuals, and the broader effect of collective death on a community constitute a resource whose significance is greater than the sum of the individual parts. This is of social impact. There is a responsibility to history that the record of these events is maintained, ordered and archived in a manner which will make this possible. Perhaps the archaeologist's final obligation to the site and its community is to ensure that this is the case.

REFERENCES

Connor, M., and Scott, D.D. (2001). Paradigms and perpetrators. *Journal of Historical Archaeology, 35*(1):1–6.

CPA (Coalition Provisional Authority) (2003). *Operational field guide.* Internal document. Baghdad: CPA.

Haglund, W.D. (2002). Recent mass graves, an introduction. In *Advances in forensic taphonomy: Method, theory and archaeological perspectives*, Haglund, W.D., and Sorg, M.H. (Eds.). Boca Raton: CRC Press, pp. 243–261.

Haglund, W.D., Connor, M., and Scott, D.D. (2001). The archaeology of contemporary mass graves. *Journal of Historical Archaeology, 35*(1):57–69.

Hoshower, L.M. (1998). Forensic archaeology and the need for flexible excavation strategies: A case study. *J. Forensic Sciences, 43*(1):53–56.

Hunter, J. R., and Cox, M. (2005). *Forensic archaeology: Advances in theory and practice.* London: Routledge.

Hunter, J.R., Karaska, M., Reddick, A., Scott, J., and Tetlow, E. (2005). *Location of mass graves using non-invasive remote sensing equipment, geophysics, and satellite imagery.* Report commissioned by the International Commission on Missing Persons (ICMP). Sarajevo: ICMP.

Hunter, J.R., Roberts, C., and Martin, A. (1996). *Studies in crime: An introduction to forensic archaeology.* London: Batsford (Reprinted 1997, by Routledge: London).

ICRC (International Committee of the Red Cross) (2003). *Explosive remnants of war.* Geneva: ICRC.

ICRC (International Committee of the Red Cross) (2004). *Operational best practices regarding the management of human remains and information on the dead by non-specialists.* Geneva: ICRC.

ICTY (International Criminal Tribunal for the former Yugoslavia) (2001). *Protocols for forensic team.* Internal document. The Hague: ICTY.

Komar, D. (2003). Lessons from Srebrenica: The contributions and limitations of physical anthropology in identifying victims of war crimes. *Journal of Forensic Science, 48*(4):713–716.

Skinner, M. (1987). Planning the archaeological recovery of evidence from recent mass graves. *Forensic Sciences International, 34*:267–287.

Skinner, M., Alempijevic, D. and Djuric-Srejic, M. (2003). Guidelines for international forensic bio-archaeology monitors of mass grave exhumations. *Forensic Science International, 134*:81–92.

Skinner, M., and Sterenberg, J. (2005). Turf wars: Authority and responsibility for the investigation of mass graves. *Forensic Science International, 151*:221–232.

Steadman, D.W., and Haglund, W.D. (2005). The scope of anthropological contributions to human rights investigations. *J. Forensic Sciences, 50*(1):23–30.

Stover, E., and Ryan, M. (2001). Breaking bread with the dead. *Journal of Historical Archaeology, 35*(1):7–25.

United Nations (1949). *Geneva Convention relative to the protection of civilian persons in time of war.* Geneva: United Nations.

United Nations (1977). *Geneva Convention: Protocol 1.* Geneva: United Nations.

United Nations (1991). *Manual on the effective prevention and investigation of extra-legal, arbitrary and summary executions* ("The Minnesota Protocol"). New York: United Nations.

Wright, R., Hanson, I., and Sterenberg, J. (2005). *The archaeology of mass graves. In Forensic archaeology: Advances in theory and practice*, Hunter, J.R., and Cox, M. (Eds.). London: Routledge, pp. 137–158.

INDEX